Refuting
Peter Singer's
Ethical Theory

Refuting
Peter Singer's
Ethical Theory

The Importance of Human Dignity

Susan Lufkin Krantz

PRAEGER

Westport, Connecticut
London

Library of Congress Cataloging-in-Publication Data

Krantz, Susan Lufkin.
  Refuting Peter Singer's ethical theory : the importance of human dignity /
Susan Lufkin Krantz.
    p. cm.
  Includes bibliographical references and index.
  ISBN 0–275–97083–3 (alk. paper)
  1. Singer, Peter, 1946– I. Title.
B5704.S554K73 2002
170′.92—dc21   2001036696

British Library Cataloguing in Publication Data is available.

Library of Congress Catalog Card Number: 2001036696
ISBN: 0–275–97083–3

First published in 2002

Praeger Publishers, 88 Post Road West, Westport, CT 06881
An imprint of Greenwood Publishing Group, Inc.
www.praeger.com

Printed in the United States of America

The paper used in this book complies with the
Permanent Paper Standard issued by the National
Information Standards Organization (Z39.48–1984).

10 9 8 7 6 5 4 3 2

This book is dedicated to
RICHARD A. GABRIEL
teacher, scholar, humanist, and dear friend

and to the memory of
RODERICK M. CHISHOLM
1916–1999
who taught us all that metaphysics still matters

I abhorred the face of man. Oh, not abhorred! they were my brethren, my fellow beings, and I felt attracted even to the most repulsive of them, as to creatures of an angelic nature and celestial mechanism. But I felt I had no right to share their intercourse. I had unchained an enemy among them, whose joy it was to shed their blood and revel in their groans.

—Mary Shelley, *Frankenstein*

They say that terror is a disease, and anyhow, I can witness that, for several years now, a restless fear has dwelt in my mind, such a restless fear as a half-tamed lion cub may feel. My trouble took the strangest form. I could not persuade myself that the men and women I met were not also another, still passably human, Beast People, animals half-wrought into the outward image of human souls, and that they would presently begin to revert, to show first this bestial mark and then that. But I have confided my case to a strangely able man, a man who had known Moreau, and seemed half to credit my story, a mental specialist—and he has helped me mightily.

—H.G. Wells, *The Island of Dr. Moreau*

We humanize each other by our willingness to *include* others within that basic fellowship—the sick, the deformed, the retarded, the old. We have not become fully human unless we recognize their humanity. It is a mark of the humane to extend its own obligations—even to a kindness toward animals.

—Gary Wills, *Under God: Religion in American Politics*

Contents

Chapter Five
Why Singer's Principle of Equal Consideration Is a Threat
to Morality and to Human Values
97

Chapter Six
On Human Dignity
119

Select Bibliography
125

Index
129

Acknowledgments

This book could not have been written without a lot of help from my friends. Prof. Joseph Spoerl first inspired me to begin thinking about the work of Peter Singer when I foolishly mentioned that I couldn't understand why he was spending a sabbatical on that topic. The more I read, though, the more I saw the importance of it. Prof. Richard Gabriel encouraged me to turn my thoughts about Singer's ethics into a book, pointing out that the time is ripe for it. Dr. Paul Gagliardi and Alison Felder Gagliardi, RN, kindly agreed to read the manuscript with a view to spotting errors in medical terminology. Professors Richard Gabriel, Benedict Guevin, Joseph Spoerl, John van Ingen, and Joseph Uemura all gave generously of their time to read earlier versions of the book, and offered many suggestions for improvement. Prof. Barbara Stahl helped me to understand better the biological issues involved. Able assistance by Lucille Murrell and Paul Taglini of the Department of Information Technology at St. Anselm College also has been much appreciated. In the end, while I take full responsibility for the errors and gaps that remain, I am hopeful that those who read the book will be prompted to think about the ethical issues of our day in light of genuinely human values, and to apply their intelligence in the very necessary project of developing a healthy moral image for the future.

Introduction

During the early centuries of the first millennium A.D., in a period now known as Late Antiquity, pagan philosophers were held in high esteem as one variety of "holy men," uniquely in touch with the gods and able to mediate divine wisdom to the common people. The ideas those philosophers propounded were often far removed from the daily realities that most people faced, yet they carried weight culturally because the philosophers themselves were so respected. Ordinary people did not consider themselves qualified to criticize the philosophers' ideas thanks to the general otherworldly aura surrounding philosophy.

Today the situation is essentially unchanged. Though we are notoriously pragmatic in the West, with highly developed technology, unprecedented reverence for the marketplace and precious little time to pursue wisdom, still we tend to feel that the thinkers among us, including academic philosophers, have a privileged access to the deeper truths. Thus even if his or her ideas are far removed from the daily realities that most people face, it is possible for a philosopher today to gain a wide audience and high respect. Ordinary people may find the philosopher's conclusions preposterous, but they do not consider themselves qualified to criticize the ideas those conclusions are based on, thanks to the general otherworldly aura surrounding philosophy.

Such is the present case of Professor Peter Singer, newly appointed Ira W. DeCamp Professor of Bioethics at Princeton University's Center for Human Values. In his version of utilitarian ethics, he has drawn conclusions that no sane person will easily accept—a newborn human infant has no more value than a snail, for instance, and a brain-damaged human being may have no more value than a cabbage—but feeling themselves unqualified to criticize the principles upon which his conclusions are based, or to find errors in his reasoning, non-philosophers have assumed that he must have a point worth heeding. Animal rights activists have been intrigued with Singer's work, and those concerned with life issues such as abortion and euthanasia have paid attention. Philosophers themselves, because of their fascination with ideas and rational argumentation, have taken Singer's views quite seriously, despite the fact that there are obvious gaps and inconsistencies in his reasoning. So lay people and professionals alike have been in awe, even though Singer's ethical theory is clearly an affront to our common humanity.

My primary purpose is to expose the basic mistake of Singer's ethical theory in such a way that the average educated person can see where Singer's theory would lead us and why we, as a society, should not want to go there. This is not to impugn Singer's character or his motives, however, in which there is indeed much to admire. He has taken seriously the pressing bio-medical issues of our day, and has championed the claims of the needy against the affluent (not only the claims of the other animals against human beings) in such a way as to remind us of St. Francis Assisi. Singer may even be a holy man (he does give one-fifth of his income to famine relief), but like many of the saints he apparently has scant regard for ordinary human attachments and therein lies the source of the error and the danger of his ethical theory. For although his basic ethical principles are not likely to occur to the ordinary person, or if they do to seem suspicious, his conclusions could well have a disastrous effect on many of our lives should they become commonly accepted. The relation between Singer's principles and his conclusions is one main topic of this book.

To examine carefully the relations between principles and the conclusions derived from them is philosophical work, but I do not intend this to be primarily a philosophical study in that narrow sense. I do not delve into the conceptual intricacies of competing ethical or meta-ethical theories, nor do I defend one theory against others. I am concerned rather to defend the dignity of our humanity against Peter Singer's ethical theory, and by extension, against any overly rationalistic ethics, a defense that should be of interest to all of us and not just to professional philosophers. Often what is of great importance to philosophers is of almost no importance at all to the intelligent non-philosopher. In teaching ethics, for example, though philosophers see all the difference in the world between a utilitarian and a Kantian, and though to a large extent my philosophical sympathies are with Kant, I actually prefer the development of a thoughtful, humanistic utilitarian to that of a rigid, legalistic Kantian. Both utilitarians and Kantians, in other words, are quite capable of regarding or disregarding real human concerns, and in the long run regard for humanity may be far more important to teacher and to student than any philosophical advantage of a given theory. So in discussing Singer's work I examine ethical principles and their consequences with a view to encouraging true humanism in ethics, but without attempting to construct or defend a complete ethical theory in the philosophical sense.

My discussion of Singer's ethical theory is organized around its basic principles, first presenting an interpretation and then offering a critique of each. There are essentially four points made by Singer that need to be addressed:[1] (1) the goal of philosophical ethics is to find a fundamental ethical principle, because our intuitions and social or religious views are inadequate; (2) moral values cannot be objective because they are not "out there" in the universe to be discovered; (3) the role of reason in ethics is to universalize our preferences so that we may transcend our personal perspective; and (4) equal consideration must be given to the interests of all sentient beings because where moral standing is concerned considerations of species membership are arbitrary and hence morally irrelevant. After examining these ideas, I focus more closely on Singer's principle of equal consideration of interests, showing how it fails as an ethical principle, what obnoxious conclusions it leads to, and ultimately how it flies in the face of what is now known about the role of the emotions in human reasoning and decision making.

Along the way I suggest in outline a humanistic alternative to Singer's ethical theory, again without involving the reader in the intricacies of philosophers' theoretical disputes and admittedly, too, without proposing a complete ethical theory of my own. I intend the philosophical sketch of a better direction for ethics to be applicable both to utilitarian and non-utilitarian theories, and to be of interest to both religious and non-religious people. Singer sees himself as an opponent of the prevailing Judeo-Christian ethos, and that may well be part of the reason why his views have seemed dangerous to some. But upon closer examination it becomes apparent that the real point at issue is not whether we shall believe in God and traditional morality, but whether we shall duly prize our common humanity. Our answer to this latter question is a matter of the gravest importance for all of us who hope to live, and to see our children's children live, in the twenty-first century. In my opinion, the human world that would result if Singer's principles were to dominate is unacceptable, though already very much in evidence at the dawn of the third millennium. Already decisions about fundamental questions concerning human life and death are being made, and policies based on those decisions are taking effect, regardless of whether they are well thought out and humane. Often the driving forces behind them are nothing more than the values of the marketplace. And if Singer's ethical principles and the conclusions drawn from them are allowed to prevail the result will be moral shipwreck, thanks to precipitous loss of respect for the dignity of human life.

NOTE

1. For this summary, and for many other insights into the work of Peter Singer I am indebted to the meticulous scholarship and astute analysis of my colleague, Professor Joseph Spoerl.

Chapter One

The Goal of Ethics

The root meaning of the word 'ethics,' as of the word 'morality,' is custom or customary behavior. Both roots, the Greek (*ethike*) and the Latin (*mos*), have as their original signification the sense of appropriateness that custom and the customary involve. Over time—both historically and within the lifetime of an individual—the overtones of 'right' and 'wrong' are added to the basic concept of the appropriate, so that for a mature civilization or person what is ethical or morally right means far more than just what counts as acceptable behavior. Anthropology studies the varieties of acceptable behavior in diverse societies, while the study of right and wrong as such is typically considered to be the province of that branch of philosophy known as ethics. The task of anthropology is clear; information must be gathered, organized, and interpreted in the manner of empirical science. This is a descriptive, factual task. The task of ethics is less clear because no amount of description of how people actually do behave will by itself yield knowledge of how they ought to behave. The knowledge sought by ethics is normative or evaluative, that is to say, not merely descriptive. Ethics functions on the non-factual plane of value, principle, and prescription, rather than on the factual plane of action and description.

Because ethics deals in the normative there is a sense in which it always transcends everyday life; thus it is no accident that through much of human history religion has played a role in ethical thought. Care must be taken, however, to avoid the hasty conclusion that ethics has ordinarily been a kind of religious thinking only recently secularized, as Peter Singer and the British philosopher Derek Parfit contend.[1] Quite possibly, the transcendent dimension in which both religion and ethics operate and find meaning is a feature of the human psyche capable of lending itself independently to both pursuits. In any event, human beings have speculated about right and wrong at least since the ancient Egyptians first believed that Pharaoh himself, the son of Ra, had the obligation to do *Maat*, or what is fitting and right.[2] Ethics to this day tries to understand what is right and good at some level of generality; that is, in a way not confined to the immediacy of individual decision making. The domain of ethics is right action and good character in general, which necessarily involves the study of ethical principles.

SINGER'S CRITIQUE OF OUR BASIC MORAL INTUITIONS

Singer sees it as the primary task of philosophical ethics to discover the fundamental ethical principle. That this should be something obscure and in need of discovery may come as a surprise to some people, however. Don't we all basically *know* what's right, and isn't the problem rather to get ourselves to *do* what's right in a tough situation?[3] But to assume that we basically know what's right is to assume that either our ethical intuitions or our moral (and perhaps religious) traditions are correct, which is precisely the point that Singer means to call into question. Many of our ordinary beliefs about right and wrong, he believes, are mistaken and ill-founded.

For instance, most of us hold as a basic ethical belief that our moral obligations to family and close friends are more binding on us, and more demanding of us, than are our moral obligations to people unrelated to us or whom we have never met. We think it a moral imperative to feed our own children, but say that those who go out of their way to feed somebody else's children, too, are acting "above and beyond the call of duty." You should put breakfast on the table for your own three-year-old; that goes without saying, and if you fail to do so you are morally remiss. But should you also contribute to UNICEF? Yes, if you can; and if you do so, that is doing more than what is morally required, and we admire you for it. But if you can contribute to UNICEF and do not, we do not normally blame you for that. Perhaps if you can afford to give to some charity or other and yet never part with a penny, we think less of you than of somebody else who does give. We may even regard the failure to give at all as wrong. Still, it is a far lesser wrong than the wrong of depriving your own children of food. Or so our ordinary moral beliefs dictate.

So much the worse for our ordinary moral beliefs, according to Singer. The very basis of preferential treatment for family and friends is flawed in that it is essentially arbitrary.[4] Those unrelated and unknown to us suffer no less from our neglect and benefit no less from our active concern; therefore ideally they should be thought to qualify for the same degree of attention as those more closely associated with us by some accident of nature or history. In other words, the preference for family and friends is a *fact* about human behavior, but according to Singer it does not have legitimate *normative* status as a claim about how things ought to be. It is as though we were to argue from the fact that two-year-olds do not want to share their toys to the normative claim that nobody should have to share things with others. But you cannot base such a normative claim on merely factual premises. In our example it would first have to be shown that two-year-olds are *right* not to want to share their toys, and presumably this cannot be done. Likewise, Singer would say, it cannot be shown to be right to give preference to family and friends; what can be shown is only that people do exhibit this preference. Moreover the preference itself can be explained on entirely non-normative grounds as an adaptation conducive to the survival of our genes; because the exigencies of evolution are no source of moral knowledge, its claim to be a fundamental moral intuition is undermined. We favor family and friends, in other words, not because it is right to do so, but because this increases our chances of successfully passing our genes on to subsequent generations. But, Singer tells us, "A biological explanation of the prevalence of kin preference undermines [its] claim" to be a self-evident principle of morality.[5]

Sociobiology, that branch of anthropology which studies human behavior as the product of the evolution of a social mammal, is a rich though flawed source of moral insight for Singer.[6] As he points out, rightly in my opinion, the fact that a strong preference or behavioral tendency can be explained by evolutionary biology does not entitle us to accept the preference or tendency as being morally right for human beings. Such an inference from what *happens to be* natural to what *ought to be* done is unwarranted. Deceptive behavior and lying, for instance, are common if not universal among human beings (and among the great apes),[7] but this does not mean that any moral code should endorse deceit. Singer draws a further conclusion, though. Not only are our moral actions (such as lying) and intuitions (such as kin preference) not validated by the findings of evolutionary biology, those findings actually serve to discredit or undermine our moral intuitions. In other words, that kin preference can be shown to have a biological basis means for Singer that it cannot serve as a moral principle. It is important to notice the argumentative move here, for one might expect the existence of a biological (factual) explanation to have an entirely neutral effect on a moral (normative) claim. But for Singer there is more to it than this.

Because we are social mammals and members of a species that has evolved over time, much of what is customary, acceptable, and right behavior for us must be seen as simply the result of natural selection. Altruistic behavior, for instance, has survival value as well as being the source of our concepts of ethical behavior.[8] Kin altruism, reciprocal altruism, and group altruism all aid us in passing on our genes because our kin, other reciprocating members of our group, and the group itself that we belong to all promote our own survival and successful reproduction as well as the safety and eventual successful reproduction of our progeny. From a purely self-interested point of view, then, it is a fact that altruistic behavior is to be recommended, and so there is no genuine moral value to be found in the altruistic behavior of social mammals, humans included. But the picture is more complicated than this; for if sociobiology were to have shown, as is often thought, that humans are basically motivated by self-interest, then we could continue to think of ethics as unaffected by sociobiological facts. The factual findings, that is to say, would have no bearing on our normative principles. Yet it turns out, as Singer notes, that "there is an evolutionary advantage in having genuine concern for others," assuming "that potential partners can see through a pretense of altruism."[9] Psychological studies show that we favor those we regard as truly caring about our welfare and are less likely to practice reciprocal altruism with egoistic phonies. This means in general, because altruism is at the root of ethics, that our moral intuitions are biologically based—"sociobiology itself can explain the existence of genuinely altruistic motivation"[10]—and thus our moral intuitions are "debunked" or shown to be suspect from the outset. As a result, Singer holds, we need to rest ethics on a different foundation, one not a product of our biology.

Edward O. Wilson, the leading exponent of sociobiological explanations in ethics, holds the hope that science, besides giving us better knowledge about the consequences of our actions, will also undermine the credibility of traditional moral principles (by showing how they have resulted from evolutionary adaptations) and provide us with new and better moral principles (thanks to the new biology of ethics).[11] To a large extent, Singer agrees especially with the critical side of this program, illustrating the need for it with his observation that kin preference is being abolished as we "expand the circle" of ethics to include all humanity (and one day, he hopes, to include all sentient beings, human and non-human).[12] Reason does not support kin preference as a moral principle because reason is on the side of impartiality,[13] and because by the use of reason we see that a moral principle is something quite different from a biological adaptation.

SINGER'S CRITIQUE OF TRADITIONAL MORALITY

Biological adaptations are also largely responsible for our beliefs about sexual morality—for instance the notorious "double standard," according to which the same level of sexual activity before marriage is considered excusable in a man (he's just "sowing wild oats") and inexcusable in a woman (she's a "slut").[14] Reproductive strategies that make sense for males do not make sense for females, which is how that got started. What appears subjectively unquestionable to those who have a given moral intuition can thus be objectively unfounded morally speaking, due to its undisputed biological origins. So we must look beyond the moral intuitions we owe to our biological history if we are to find the fundamental ethical principle.

But as Singer points out:

It is not only biological explanations which have the effect of debunking accepted ethical principles. To complete the process, we would have to explore the history of the ethical beliefs of our own particular society. Then we would find relics of our cultural history to place alongside the relics of our evolutionary history. For instance, the Western principle of the sanctity of human life.[15]

The relics of our cultural history include outmoded religious traditions, economic or social circumstances of the past, and prudery about sexuality and bodily functions.[16] Their effect is to make us subjectively confident of moral principles and judgments that have no genuinely moral foundation at all. The result of this is that we enshrine historical accidents as inviolable moral law.

One serious issue which Singer sees as illustrating the inadequacy of our traditional moral judgments is the medical definition of death. According to Singer's account,[17] the medical definition of death, and consequently traditional moral norms about taking human life, have been under pressure from two sides: (1) from medical advances which have made it possible to maintain a patient in a persistent vegetative state for a long period of time (the record for such survival without a respirator was over thirty-seven years in 1981, thanks to tube feeding, hydration, and antibiotics); and (2) from the demand for organs and tissues to prolong the lives of otherwise healthy patients who can be saved or whose quality of life can be meaningfully enhanced by transplants. Traditionally, death had been defined as the cessation of cardiopulmonary function.[18] This was in fact a nineteenth-century resolution of difficulties inherited from an earlier period during which it became apparent that sometimes people had inadvertently been buried alive (they revived in their coffins, or later exhumations showed evidence of the allegedly deceased having attempted to claw their way out of the tomb). Laws were passed to ensure that the buried were truly dead, and some eighteenth century physicians held that putrefaction is the only conclusive evidence of death.[19] With the development of the modern stethoscope, however, it was more possible to detect a heartbeat in difficult cases, and since heartbeat and respiration are closely interdependent, the criterion of death became their absence. Evidently the public then relaxed as concern about ghoulish prospects of being buried alive subsided. In our day, medical advances have again had an effect on our understanding of death, but in the reverse direction. Because we now have the capacity to save patients with certain kinds of conditions by means of organ and tissue transplants, and because we know enough about brain function to be fairly sure when a patient in a persistent vegetative (or non-cognitive) state will not recover consciousness, the question arises of what to do when an organ from a patient in a persistent vegetative state would save the life of a patient who, if treated, will be able to continue conscious life.

In 1968, when the cessation of cardiopulmonary function was still the commonly accepted medical definition of death, steps were taken to come up with a new definition in order to cope with this kind of situation. The Harvard Brain Death Committee sought "to define irreversible coma as a new criterion for death."[20] The committee cited two reasons for establishing a new criterion: first, the burden placed on families, hospitals and society by comatose patients; and second, the need to obtain organs for transplantation. As Singer points out, this was a pragmatic move, a stipulative definition in order to gain certain advantages, and not at all a disinterested discovery about the truth concerning biological death. In the intervening decades we have come to accept some form of "brain death" as constituting the death of the human organism for all practical purposes, but this is not to say that there is any clear, general understanding of what this means, nor that there are no problems remaining. The President's Commission of 1981 insisted on a criterion of "whole brain death"; that is to say the cessation of function in all three main areas of the brain, the cerebrum with its cortex, the cerebellum, and the brainstem which controls non-conscious life functions. Their argument was that heartbeat, respiration, and brain function are intimately interrelated in such a way that the old definition of death in terms of the cessation of cardiopulmonary function can be regarded as the equivalent of whole brain death. Thus the traditional understanding of death, though enhanced by further knowledge of brain function, is not essentially altered by its replacement with the terminology of whole brain death. Of course, the irreversibly comatose, those in a persistent vegetative (or non-cognitive) state, are not dead by either the traditional definition or the whole brain death definition. Whether unaided or with the intervention of medical technology, these patients continue to have heartbeat and respiration, and they have partial brain function (mainly limited to the brainstem).

But in fact it is possible for patients with no brainstem function to survive for a period of time. Thus it sometimes happens that a patient in persistent vegetative state whose organs are needed for another patient will be taken off life support and allowed to go into cardiac arrest. Transplant team physicians and nurses then wait for two minutes after cardiac arrest occurs before removing the organs, but while removing the organs they do not treat the body as though it were a corpse (even though legally, by the whole brain criterion, it is) since there is a chance the body could revive.[21] What can revive, however, is not really dead. In cases like this, organs are being removed from living human bodies that happen to satisfy the legal criteria of death. The brain dead are known frequently to respond to surgical incision with increased heart rate and blood pressure. Not only that, but all the legally brain dead who are otherwise living (whether by the aid of life support, or unaided) have hormonal activity of which the brain itself is the only source. At the dawn of the twenty-first century, then, it seems that we are back to square one in terms of staving off the horrible prospect of being buried alive! As Robert Truog notes, "The thought of burying or cremating a breathing individual, even if unconscious, would be unthinkable for many people, creating a barrier to acceptance of [the higher brain definition of death] into public policy."[22]

The question of what to do about this admits of two main kinds of answer: either (1) it is time, despite public opinion, to abandon the whole brain definition of death in favor of a higher brain definition; or (2) it is time to admit that sometimes it is morally permissible to kill living human beings, for instance, when they have no hope of recovering consciousness so far as we know, and somebody else is in need of their organs. Peter Singer rejects the first alternative as dishonest and counterintuitive.[23] Instead, he recommends that we bite the bullet and admit that our traditional moral principles concerning the taking of human life are outworn and in need of replacement. It would be wrong, in other words, to pretend that some organ donors are actually dead when their organs are taken, if all ordinary indications are to the contrary. Better to admit that sometimes we have to kill people for the greater good.

Traditional ethical systems in the West have answered questions about the morality of taking human life by relying on the principle of the sanctity of human life. It is this principle that Singer claims we must now abandon under pressure from medical advances and improved understanding of primate biology and behavior. The sanctity of human life had been grounded in the belief that human beings are unique in the known universe, especially due to their powers of reasoning and speech. "Man is the rational animal," according to the traditional philosophical definition, which held that reason is what separates us from the other animals. But now that we know more about the other primates, especially the great apes—gorillas, orangutans, and chimpanzees—we must relinquish our claim to be unique. Singer advances essentially two reasons for this: (1) the great apes are able to do things that had been thought uniquely human—they use tools, learn American sign language, make jokes, and tell lies; and (2) genetically the great apes are very close to us, especially chimpanzees with whom we share 98.4% of our DNA.[24] These considerations should lead us to realize that our former claim to being created uniquely "in the image of God" is unwarranted and thus not an adequate basis for moral judgments.

Moreover, according to Singer, our "speciesist" belief in human superiority and uniqueness is analogous to, and just as morally reprehensible as, racist claims of superiority and consequent privilege. Just as the races of mankind are now known to be fundamentally equal, such that racial discrimination is no longer socially acceptable while interracial marriage now is, so in the future we must be prepared to give equal consideration to the interests of chimpanzees and other great apes. Even "the possibility of human and chimpanzee interbreeding cannot be ruled out."[25] As we "expand the circle" of ethical concern beyond our family, neighbors, ethnic group, and race, so as moral enlightenment grows, in Singer's view, we shall be drawn to expand the circle beyond our species.

This will require a moral revolution not unlike the Copernican revolution in physics brought about by the realization that the planets form a heliocentric, and not a geocentric, system. Likewise until now our ethical universe has been unduly focussed on human beings; a shift in paradigm will lead us to see the most important moral issues of our day in a completely new light. For Singer this means especially that we will be moved to give equal consideration to the interests of all sentient creatures, and that we will revise our standards about the termination of human life as we begin to see that personhood—the morally significant feature of individuals who may be thought to have a right to life, other things being equal—is not confined to the human species. As it turns out, all animals have moral standing, in virtue of being sentient. But only some human beings are persons, as are many non-human animals, and only persons have an interest in continuing to exist in the future.[26]

SINGER'S SEARCH FOR THE FUNDAMENTAL ETHICAL PRINCIPLE

From Singer's point of view, then, it is clear that the ethical tradition we have received is ill-founded, inadequate, and in need of replacement.

It is ill-founded both at the level of basic moral intuition, and at the level of moral judgment based on principle. For our basic moral intuitions are derived from our nature as biological organisms which have evolved under circumstances that happen to have favored the development of the basic intuitions that we happen to have. In other words, there is nothing inherently moral about the intuitions that appear to us to be moral, for instance the intuition that we have stronger moral obligations to our close family and friends than we do to others. This is a feeling and a tendency that has survival value, nothing more. Similarly, the principle of the sanctity of human life, and moral judgments based on it regarding life and death decisions, are suspect because derived from a social and religious tradition that represents a false worldview.

Human beings are not the center of the ethical universe; moreover, it is morally wrong to think so.

In both cases—in the critique of moral intuition, and in the critique of moral principle and judgment—reason is decisive for Singer, because it shows that the evolutionary basis of intuition, and the cultural basis of moral principle and judgment, are inadequate. Kin preference is not rational; it is a mere accident of evolutionary advantage. The sanctity of human life as such is not a rational principle because there is no rational line to be drawn between human life and non-human life, as the case of the chimpanzees shows.

Reason also makes it clear that our traditional ethics is not working. The disputes concerning the definition of death, including the redefinition of death in order to permit the removal of organs for transplant and the dilemmas caused by the "dead donor rule,"[27] show that we need a new understanding of the permissibility of taking human life. This cuts to the very quick of society's understanding of ethics, and sharply points out the need for a new fundamental ethical principle. For Singer, ethics is largely the search for such a principle, grounded in reason and free of the biological and cultural baggage of the old ethical paradigm.

REPLY TO SINGER ON MORAL INTUITION

Singer is right to advocate examination of our moral intuitions and principles. Surely intelligent moral thinking is a legitimate goal of philosophical ethics, and if our moral intuitions were mindless, knee-jerk reactions rooted in our evolutionary biology and nothing more, then we should seriously consider their replacement. As we have seen, Singer believes this to be true of such moral intuitions as the belief, founded in kin preference, that our moral obligations are greater to those who are near and dear to us than to those we have never met. Though he rejects the claim of sociobiology to produce a "biology of ethics" (an improvement over the old ethics), because that would involve deriving values from facts—the so-called "naturalistic fallacy"— still he accepts the power of sociobiological findings to debunk our basic moral intuitions. This seems to me to be a mistake.

Consider kin preference. It is normal for human beings to favor their near relatives' interests over those of human beings who are more remote, and even over their own interests sometimes, as instances of altruistic behavior show. Granted, from the fact alone that this is normal, no normative or evaluative claims can be derived. However, just as it is a mistake to reduce values to facts, so it is also a mistake to bleed the human nature factor out of ethics entirely. If sociobiology does nothing else, it certainly provides abundant lore about what is natural behavior for the human animal. To assume, as Singer seems to do, that we discredit a moral intuition by showing it to be natural is to go far beyond what sociobiological findings could ever possibly justify—as surely so as it would be to imagine that sociobiological findings amount to an endorsement of an ethical intuition. But neither endorsement nor debunking follow from the sociobiological facts. What follows is just that in dealing with human beings we are dealing with animals of a certain type, for whom certain behaviors are natural in a general way. Kin preference may be seen as one of these behaviors. The moral intuition about greater obligation to one's kin is a moral belief, a normative claim, neither supported nor discredited by the facts.

Two examples may illustrate this. One, mentioned earlier, is the propensity of two-year-old human beings to resist sharing their toys. From the fact that they rarely share, or do so reluctantly, nothing follows about whether they should share or not. We say they should share; but that's a normative, moral claim, not a factual one. A second illustration is marital fidelity. Suppose no more than 4% of spouses are unfaithful in the United States in a given year. From the fact that the vast majority are faithful, nothing would follow about whether they should be faithful or not. We say monogamy is a good thing; but that's a normative, moral claim, not a factual one. Suppose somebody came along, as several did in the 1960s and 1970s, and declared that truly enlightened adults would share their spouses with one another. The vast majority, over time at least, would conclude that this was nutty, a false moral claim that flies in the face of ordinary moral intuition. And the vast majority would be right about the moral side of the question, whether they subsequently took up wife-swapping or not! The logical independence of fact and value is of ultimate importance for clear moral thinking. Singer is, of course, a highly respected moral thinker and I would never suggest that he is unaware of this distinction; but I do believe he makes a mistake with respect to it when he assumes that the facts of sociobiology tell us anything at all about which of our moral intuitions are incorrect.

Part of the difficulty here is the whole question of the relation between biology and psychology in human beings. Biology is a purely factual realm, whereas psychology comprises both factual and normative elements. This is true even if John Searle is right, as I think he is, to hold that consciousness is a biological phenomenon.[28] For though we are conscious thanks to our brain physiology, once conscious in the way that non-infant human beings are normally conscious we dwell in a realm that partly transcends the factual, the physiological, the empirical, and even to some extent the real. How this is possible is a topic far beyond the scope of this study. That it is actual is a fact we deny at our peril. Whenever we think of things that might exist but do not, as we all do many times daily, or of courses of action that should be taken but are not, or even simply of the quality of our own experience as we "step back" from it, we acquire a bit of transcendence and become capable of several varieties of peculiarly human experience—love, aesthetic delight, contemplation of nature and ourselves, ethical thinking, religion, fantasy, fiction, art. Concerning aesthetic judgment, for instance, sociobiology can tell us what kind of animal it is that creates or admires a painting, and so forth, but nothing sociobiology can tell us about it debunks art. Likewise concerning morality, sociobiology does no debunking of intuitions—it is just out of its dimension at that level of the moral realm.

To illustrate this let us return briefly to Singer's example of the double standard in sexual morality, but setting aside the question whether that standard is justified. A variety of claims could be made at the level of biology and evolution; none of them would touch the ordinary human experiences of lust and love, for these are psychological, subjective, personal, and imbued with a rich set of qualities that no hormonal or population-biological analysis can come close to capturing. This will be true in spades for the far more complicated phenomena of jealousy and reprobation involved in the double standard. To understand it you would do better to read a novel than to take up a textbook of sociobiology. Human experience is psychological.

This holds for kin preference, too, and for the perceived moral obligation to favor our kin. In order to show that our moral intuitions in this area are incorrect it would have to be shown not just that the behavior involved is not conducive to the greatest happiness of the greatest number,[29] but also that the psychological bonds of kinship—special love for mother, father, siblings, children—are perverse. But this cannot be done. It cannot be done on the basis of facts (about who might benefit from our abandonment of kin preference), because nothing normative follows merely from the facts. And it cannot be done on the basis of values because it is an intuition and hence for human beings a basis and source of value from which other values are derived but which itself does not derive from a more fundamental value. A human being who prefers strangers to kin, in other words, is not normal. If somebody deliberately saved a stranger from a burning building instead of his mother, willfully ignoring her screams, we would know he came from a dysfunctional family, to say the least. To undermine or debunk our basis for knowing this is to strike at the very foundation of morality, not in a constructive way as Singer claims, but destructively. Take this away and there is no human morality left.

REPLY TO SINGER ON TRADITIONAL MORALITY

Besides moral intuitions at the very basic level of kin preference, we also inherit social and cultural norms and a system of moral principles and judgments grounded in them. Again, Singer is right to recommend that we examine these; moral thinking requires reflection and is the antithesis of blind obedience. But Singer's critique of our traditional morality is largely unjustified in my opinion. As we have seen, he regards many of our moral principles, and the judgments based on them, as historical accidents, consequences of outmoded religious systems, past social and economic circumstances, and the like. Let us return to the discussion of the definition of death as a prime example.

In a 1993 contribution to the *Hastings Center Report*, Robert M. Veatch expresses some surprise that there should be such a lengthy debate in our society over the three competing definitions of death—heart-oriented, whole brain-oriented, and higher brain-oriented definitions. But, as he observes:

We have been fighting over the question of who has moral standing as a full member of the human moral community, a matter that forces on us some of the most basic questions of human existence: the relation of mind and body, the rights of religious and philosophical minorities, and the meaning of life itself.[30]

The debate has continued, then, because as a society we are ambivalent about the "most basic questions of human existence." The principle of the sanctity of human life, which had formerly guided our thinking on these topics, is now under fire as Singer notes. In an age of increasing secularization it might be thought that this is only to be expected, but that assumes the sanctity of human life to be a religious idea. While it may play a role in religion (not in all religions, though), it is not a religious but rather a moral idea in my opinion, perhaps *the* moral idea. In attacking it, Singer is not just aiming to overthrow traditional ethics; he is undermining ethics itself. For ethics is a human phenomenon that involves placing value on the human as such; this is why the normative is not reducible to the factual, why values and facts are so often in conflict,

why we find no support in the wider physical universe for our preference for human beings, and why we cling to this preference nevertheless. We are moral beings; we are human.

In proposing that death be redefined in order to facilitate the pro-
curement of organs for transplant, the Harvard Committee took a giant step in the direction of replacing human values with the values of
the marketplace. Though Singer rightly sees through to the essential
cowardice of defining the living as dead so that we may not feel bad
about what we do to them, his own solution of declaring in general that
it is alright to kill innocent human beings under certain circumstances
serves the organ business no less effectively. In other words, if there is a
shortage of organs for transplant and a potential source of organs—in
live anencephalic neonates, and in the irreversibly comatose—it looks
as though the organs can be obtained either by the sneaky route (rede-
fining death) or by the direct route (legitimizing certain murders). But
either way the commodity is brought to market.

Singer knows very well that business values are the antithesis of human moral values, and writes eloquently on the subject as it impinges
on our treatment of animals in his well-known work, *Animal Liberation*.[31] Why then does he abandon the principle of the sanctity of human life? Essentially because he imagines there to be a higher principle
which obviates it; that is to say, according to Singer, just as regard for
human beings in general is a moral principle which shows racism to be
wrong, so regard for sentient beings in general is a moral principle
which shows "speciesism" to be wrong.[32] Part of his strategy in arguing
for his thesis is to show that human beings are not, in fact, unique. The
boundaries of our species are unclear, he says, as we have seen, and the
traits we take to be peculiarly human are in fact shared with non-human
species. The other part of his strategy is simply to emphasize the analogy that he sees between racism and speciesism, in order to persuade us
that the one is just as much an evil as the other. But are either of these
strategies justified?

Is it really true that the boundaries of the human species are unclear,
and that none of our attributes are peculiarly human? In appealing to
the 1.6% difference in DNA between us and the "other chimpanzees,"
Singer is assuming that a quantitative analysis accounts for the qualitative facts, something that is not at all necessarily true. He infers that because the percentage difference is slight, therefore the real difference is
slight. But that does not follow. Why not infer, instead, that the great
and obvious difference is clearly not accounted for on a quantitative basis, in other words, that percentages of DNA tell us very little about the

qualitative differences between species? As a matter of fact, it is quite possible for species with a high percentage of DNA in common to differ sharply from one another. This is because so-called "gene expression" is also an important factor. Thus the very same gene for eye development (called "eyeless") exists in humans and mice, as well as in fruit flies and squids, that is to say, the identical gene exists in mammals, arthropods, and mollusks. But the resulting eye development is vastly different from species to species; the gene is expressed differently in the eye of a fly than in the human eye. Likewise, the genes for brain development are expressed very differently in human beings and in chimpanzees.[33]

As we have seen, Singer suggests that humans and chimpanzees might interbreed. That's an abstract speculation. Setting aside what we know about what some desperate human beings have done with sheep and goats, how many dates do we really think a chimpanzee could get using an internet dating service if he or she included an unretouched photograph?[34] Human beings have published articles on the behavior of the great apes, and much has been learned about them, which should certainly have the effect, if nothing else, of encouraging us to treat them humanely. But how many articles have the great apes written about us? How many chimpanzees are trying to teach their languages to human beings? How many gorillas care about the human beings starving in sub-Saharan Africa? How many orangutans are concerned about human beings on death row in Texas?

One does not need to believe that human beings are created in the image of God in order to realize that human beings are unique and special, *from a human point of view*. As we shall see, Singer wants us to abandon the human point of view in favor of the "point of view of the universe."[35] But this would spell the death of ethics and of every human value. We are animals of a distinct species; we recognize and are attracted to each other. So far from being a moral abomination like racism, the moral insight first gained by the ancient Egyptians that human beings are all equally bound by the principles of justice and fairness to other human beings[36] is an insight so fundamental to ethics that without it there would be no such thing. To call this "speciesism" is more than an abuse of language, though that too; it is a surreptitious coup, an overthrow of morality on allegedly moral grounds.

Mankind *is* at the center of human ethics, necessarily so. There is no Copernican revolution in the offing, as Singer foresees, for either humanity will retain its central position in the ethical universe, or else human ethics will come to an end and the values of the marketplace or some other horror will fill the vacuum. It is preposterous to suppose otherwise, as though human beings could transcend their very humanity and become, unlike any other species of animal on earth, advocates of a position inherently not their own. This is not to say that we should be cruel to creatures outside our species; far from it, for that would be beneath us. But if I am kind to the other animals, it is not because I think they are human, too, as though there were no line between species—rather it is because *I* am human that I want to treat the other animals humanely. Likewise, if there are people on Mars, as Brentano says, we should wish them well.[37] But the foundation for all ethical concern is our very human concern for one another. This is an interpersonal, face-to-face thing, fundamentally—thus the adage, "charity begins at home." "Expanding the circle" of ethical concern, in the way that Singer recommends, by abandoning our preference for our own kind is moral suicide.

REPLY TO SINGER ON THE FUNDAMENTAL ETHICAL PRINCIPLE

Singer seeks to replace our intense personal attachment to one another—to family, friends, ethnic group, and species—by a more rationally acceptable principle. Reason, in his view, will illuminate for us a better basic moral principle than the moral intuitions and principles that have been transmitted to us by the accidents of evolutionary biology and history. He seeks to replace our human ethics with a non-human, universalized ethics which will result from the long-overdue paradigm shift in which the human is displaced by the sentient as the criterion of being a bearer of moral value. Reasonable as this sounds when he is inveighing against mistreatment of non-human animals and against narrow-minded, reactionary moral systems of the past, it is not reasonable at all in terms of the real goals of ethical thinking. For ethics seeks above all to humanize us, but this cannot be done by subordinating the human to an allegedly "higher" principle, no matter how rational that principle may be. In chapter four we will examine Singer's candidate for the highest principle of morality. Here, however, my purpose is somewhat more basic, namely, to call into question the very project of seeking a principle beyond the intuitively obvious ethical principle of regard for human beings as such. Whatever principle we pick, if we go beyond the ethical regard for human beings as such, we will end by subordinating human concerns to the principle. Thus, for instance, the Nazis notoriously subordinated individual human welfare to the grand project of promoting the Aryan race. Centuries before,

Plato had explored the pros and cons of creating a utopia in which the wise would rule by nature. Whether Plato's treatment is serious or facetious, the upshot is the same: imposing a rational ideal of perfection on human society is the surest way to implement the most inhuman of social institutions. What is wrong with the guardians of the state having wives in common, their children unknown to them and raised in giant "rearing pens," if this would lead to a more harmonious society in the long run?[38] The answer is simple: it's inhuman.

And it's inhuman no matter how many philosophical arguments support it, and no matter how rational it appears *prima facie*. Singer's search for the fundamental ethical principle, riding roughshod over kin preference and the sanctity of human life, has all the earmarks of a utopian scheme that will end in disaster. Not that he is wrong about everything; far from it. He is right to point out that our treatment of animals is unconscionable, right to point out that we ought to have more concern about human suffering in the third world, right to point out that morality gives meaning to life, and right to insist that the values promoted in Western culture today are empty and destructive in many instances.[39] That having been said, his proposed solution is a potential nightmare.

The cure for inhuman behavior towards human and non-human animals, the remedy for a value system gone off-track, and the key to the meaning of life is not to transcend the human and subordinate it to a "higher" principle but rather to emphasize, to empower, and to enhance whatever is distinctively human, precisely because it is human. There is no need to justify this by some further principle, and there is no need to prove that human beings have characteristics that no other species shares or ever could share. For the value and the uniqueness of human beings are grounded in their very being and not reducible to any quantitative facts about them (1.6% of DNA) nor to any qualitative features such that their loss would involve the loss of human value (for instance, artistic ability or facility with language or even "normal" intelligence). Human beings have an intrinsic value *to other human beings* (regardless of whether we amount to anything in the ultimate history of evolution or in the grand scheme of the cosmos), and this value is directly tied to our being identifiable members of an identifiable species. We recognize our own kind, and to the extent that we are ethical we value them accordingly.

In my opinion, the failure to understand this is at the heart of proposals by Singer and others to devise new rules of ethics in the face of advances in medicine and other pressures of modern life. The perceived need either to redefine death or to revamp ethics when questions are posed about harvesting organs for transplant is essentially an inability to perceive humanity in certain kinds of extreme situations. Neither live anencephalic neonates nor the irreversibly comatose are non-human— let alone dead, in the cases that have attracted attention. It is precisely because they are human (and alive) that moral questions surrounding their fate have the power to cause anguish. And the day that anguish is defused will be the day that we descend to new depths of inhumanity, which is why I regard Singer's ethics as a potential nightmare. Any ethical system that relieves normal human moral anguish by application of a rational formula for decision-making is apt to deprive us of our dignity. As the anxiety lifts we will see that its cause is gone; namely, the belief that human life has intrinsic moral value. The belief was mistaken in any event, Singer would claim. Perhaps from some non-human point of view it is.

But I am claiming that moral value is grounded in our perception of ourselves as human, and this raises the important question of whether this perception and the value based upon it can be objectively justified. In one sense, it can be, based on work by Antonio Damasio and others[40] which shows that rational decision-making is intimately connected with emotion. That is to say, apparently a normally functioning human brain reasons by way of making decisions based on feeling at certain junctures, and not purely by rational elaboration of the possible courses of action. Those like Phineas Gage who suffer damage to an area of the brain involved in the production of emotion retain the ability to reason and to calculate (to deduce and to infer), but lack the ability to come to a conclusion, especially in questions involving day to day living and in-terpersonal attachments. In light of findings such as this, it may well be argued that a human being who did not have a healthy emotional life involving close personal attachments would not be able to make ratio-nal decisions effectively. Thus if we bred kin preference and "speciesism" out of human consciousness, we might end up with a lot of decision-impaired, dysfunctional people, rather than an enlightened moral universe as Singer anticipates.

In fact, I think something like this is probably true, and I will return to the topic later in chapter five. At this point, however, we face the more philosophical question of how moral value can be grounded in subjective perception and judgment. That is to say, if it is true in the fac-tual sense that humanity is not at the center of the universe, that human beings are in effect "the third [species of] chimpanzee,"[41] that there are no distinguishing features separating us from other sentient creatures whose pleasure and pain ought therefore to count for as much as ours do, and that killing an innocent human being can be justified when the benefits to others warrant it and the life of the individual involved has lost quality below a sufficient level, then how can anybody possibly claim that the old ideas of human dignity and the sanctity of human life are anything more than subjective prejudices that fly in the face of the facts?

The grounding of moral value in our subjective perception of the value of humanity is perfectly legitimate, in my view. But how can this be defended? Singer also finds that there is a subjective source of moral value, and he rejects objective sources. The source of our knowledge of moral value, to which we now turn, is the subject of chapter two.

NOTES

1. See Derek Parfit, *Reasons and Persons* (Oxford: Clarendon Press, 1984), pp. 453–454. Parfit concludes that in future centuries, "There could clearly be higher achievements in the struggle for a wholly just world-wide community. And there could be higher achievements in all of the Arts and Sciences. But the progress could be greatest in what is now the least advanced of these Arts or Sciences. This, I have claimed, is Non-Religious Ethics. Belief in God, or in many gods, prevented the free development of moral reasoning . . . Non-Religious Ethics is at a very early stage." See also Peter Singer, *How Are We to Live: Ethics in an Age of Self-Interest* (Amherst, NY: Prometheus Books, 1995), pp. 14–15. Singer goes so far as to claim, "It is only since about 1960 that many people have systematically studied non-religious ethics." One wonders what the ancients thought they were up to, both Egyptians and Greeks. Surely Plato and Aristotle did not view their ethical thinking as inherently religious. And Socrates, moral thinker *par excellence*, was put to death for alleged impiety—hardly a religious credential.

2. See Richard A. Gabriel, *Gods of Our Fathers: The Memory of Egypt in Judaism and Christianity* (Westport, CT: Greenwood Press, 2001), especially chapter one, "The Dawn of Conscience." See also J.H. Breasted, *Development of Religion and Thought in Ancient Egypt* (New York: Harper and Row, 1959) [reprint of the 1912 edition by Charles Scribner's Sons], especially Lecture VI, "The Emergence of the Moral Sense—Moral Worthiness and the Hereafter—Scepticism and the Problem of Suffering"; Jaroslav Cerny, *Ancient Egyptian Religion* (Westport CT: Greenwood Press, 1952); Siegfried Morenz, *Egyptian Religion*, trans. Ann E. Keep (Ithaca, New York: Cornell University Press, 1973) [originally published under the title, *Aegyptische Religion*, W. Kohlhammer GmbH., 1960]; and *Religion in Ancient Egypt*, ed. Byron E. Shafer, with contributions by John Baines, Leonard

H. Lesko, David P. Silverman (Ithaca, New York: Cornell University Press, 1991).

3. With reference to his *Foundations of the Metaphysics of Morals*, Immanuel Kant wrote that, "A critic [Gottlob August Tittel] who wished to say something against that work really did better than he intended when he said that there was no new principle of morality in it but only a new formula. Who would want to introduce a new principle of morality and, as it were, be its inventor, as if the world had hitherto been ignorant of what duty is or had been thoroughly wrong about it?" See the Preface to the *Critique of Practical Reason and Other Writings in Moral Philosophy*, trans., ed., and intro., Lewis White Beck (Chicago: Chicago University Press, 1949) p. 123.

4. See, among other sources, Singer, "The Singer Solution to World Poverty: A Contentious Ethicist Explains Why Your Taste for Foie Gras is Starving Children," *New York Times Magazine*, 5 September 1999, pp. 59–63.

5. Singer, "Ethics and Sociobiology," *Zygon*, vol. 19, no. 2 (June, 1984), 141–158, p. 151. See also Singer's *The Expanding Circle: Ethics and Sociobiology* (New York: Farrar, Straus & Giroux, 1981), p. 53 and p. 69, "If we come to see specific rules of ethics as biological adaptations resulting from our evolutionary history, we may cease to regard those ethical rules as morally absolute or self-evidently certain."

6. See Singer, *The Expanding Circle*, p. ix and pp. 167–173. Singer's view is that we gain insight into ethics by seeing it as an outgrowth of group altruism observable in the behavior of social animals generally and human beings in particular. Then we can advance by application of reason to weed out undesirable moral intuitions and behaviors and breed in better ones (under cultural pressures).

7. See for instance, "The Case for the Personhood of Gorillas," by Francine Patterson and Wendy Gordon, and "Language and the Orangutan: The Old 'Person' of the Forest," by H. Lyn White Miles, in *The Great Ape Project: Equality Beyond Humanity*, eds. Paola Cavalieri and Peter Singer (New York: St. Martin's, 1993). Patterson and Gordon cite, among quite a few traits that should lead us to admit that Koko the lowland gorilla is a person, the fact that "she lies to avoid the consequences of her own misbehavior." (p. 58) Apparently Chantek the orangutan also tells lies (p. 48). While I have no quarrel with the claim that Koko, or Chantek, is a person, I disagree with Singer in that I hold it is morally significant that Koko is not human.

8. See Singer, *The Expanding Circle*, chapter 2, "The Biological Basis of Ethics," pp. 23–53. For this discussion Singer cites especially the work of Wilson and Westermark. See E. O. Wilson, *On Human Nature* (Cambridge: Harvard University Press, 1978), p. 48, and Edward Westermark, *The Origin and Development of the Moral Ideas* (London: Macmillan, 1908), chapter 23.

9. *The Expanding Circle*, pp. 44–45. Singer cites psychological research by Robert Trivers in "The Evolution of Reciprocal Altruism," *The Quarterly Review of Biology*, 46 (1971), pp. 48–49.

10. *The Expanding Circle*, p. 45.

11. See E. O. Wilson, *Sociobiology: The New Synthesis* (Cambridge: Belknap Press of Harvard University Press, 1975), Part III, ch. 27.

12. This is the principle of the equal consideration of interests discussed in chapter four.

13. See *The Expanding Circle*, p. 101.

14. Singer, "Ethics and Sociobiology," (1984), p. 154.

15. *The Expanding Circle*, p. 71.

16. Singer, "Sidgwick and Reflective Equilibrium," *The Monist*, 58 (1974), p. 516.

17. See Singer, *Rethinking Life and Death: The Collapse of our Traditional Ethics* (New York: St. Martin's Press, 1994; St. Martin's Griffin, 1996), Chapter Two, "How Death Was Redefined," pp. 20–37.

18. Singer quotes *Black's Law Dictionary*, fourth edition (St. Paul MN: West Publishing Company, 1968): "DEATH. The cessation of life; the ceasing to exist; defined by physicians as a total stoppage of the circulation of the blood, and a cessation of the animal and vital functions consequent thereupon, such as respiration, pulsation, etc." See p. 21, *Rethinking Life and Death*.

19. See *Ethical Issues in Modern Medicine*, ed. John D. Arras and Bonnie Steinbock (Mountainview CA: Mayfield Press, 1999), pp. 143–169. An abridged version of the President's Commission report is included, pp. 143–151; the original source is *Defining Death: A Report on the Medical, Legal and Ethical Issues in the Determination of Death*, President's Commission for the Study of Ethical Problems in Medicine and Biomedical and Behavioral Research (Washington, D.C.: U.S. Government Printing Office, 1981). Alex Capron, executive director of the commission is responsible for the idea, mentioned below, that whole brain death is the equivalent of cardiopulmonary death.

20. See *Rethinking Life and Death*, part one, chapter 2, "How Death Was Redefined," pp. 20–37.

21. See Robert D. Truog, "Is It Time to Abandon Brain Death?" *Hastings Center Report*, Vol. 27, No.1, Jan./Feb. 1997, 29–37, in *Ethical Issues in Modern Medicine*, pp. 160–169. The protocol described here was followed at the University of Pittsburgh at the time this article was written. Our ambivalence about it is traceable to ambiguities inherent in the concepts of brain death generally, and higher brain death in particular, according to Truog.

22. See Truog, "Is it Time to Abandon Brain Death?" p. 165. Truog suggests that if we adopted a higher brain definition of death, organs could be removed under anaesthetic (from live, anencephalic neonates—infants born

without brains—and others), and "lethal injections" could be administered
before the brain dead are buried or cremated.

   23. See *Rethinking Life and Death*, part I, chapter 3, especially pp.
50–51. See also, Robert D. Truog, "Is it Time to Abandon Brain Death?"
Truog also advocates the second option, namely the moral permissibility of
killing innocent human beings, but concedes, "The most difficult challenge
for this proposal would be to gain acceptance of the view that killing may
sometimes be a justifiable necessity for procuring transplantable organs" (p.
169). His point is that even with the enforcement of principles of nonmale-
ficence and consent, people would fear abuses. But he suggests "only by
abandoning the concept of brain death is it possible to adopt a definition of
death that is valid for all purposes, while separating questions of organ donation from dependence on the life/death dichotomy" (p. 168). Singer is not
alone in adopting this line of argument.

   24. Singer, *Rethinking Life and Death*, p. 177.

   25. Singer, *Rethinking Life and Death*, p. 180. This observation comes at
the end of a detailed discussion of the difficulty of delineating the species
Homo sapiens (pp. 169–180). The Swedish biologist, Carl Linneaus, apparently felt pressured to put humans in a different genus from the apes, although he could think of no legitimate scientific reason to do so. In light of
recent discoveries about DNA, we now know not only that humans and
chimpanzees differ by only 1.6%, but also that chimpanzees and gorillas differ
by 2.3%, which means that we are closer to the chimps than the gorillas are.
Thus Richard Dawkins of Oxford and Jared Diamond of UCLA have suggested that we rush in where Linnaeus feared to tread and classify chimpanzees in the genus *homo*. The two species of chimpanzee, then, instead of
being *Pan troglodytes* and *Pan paniscus*, would be *Homo troglodytes* and
Homo paniscus, making *Homo sapiens* the third chimpanzee. Richard
Dawkins has made a study of "ring species," or pairs of related species which,
though they may never interbreed now, nevertheless once did interbreed
with the perhaps now extinct intermediaries between them. Human beings
and chimpanzees are such a pair, i.e., potentially members of a ring species.

   26. By "person" Singer means an individual that is self-aware and future-oriented (capable of seeing itself as persisting in time). This is roughly
the definition of "person" proposed by John Locke (1632–1704). Singer rejects the ancient definition of a person as "an individual substance of a rational nature," proposed by Boethius (480–524). Singer has reasons for
preferring a definition in terms of psychological attributes; I discuss this topic
later. For Singer's discussion, see *Rethinking Life and Death*, pp. 180–183.

   27. See Truog, "Is It Time to Abandon Brain Death?" in *Ethical Issues in
Modern Medicine*, p. 164.

   28. See John Searle, *Mind, Language, Society*, chapter two, "Mind as a Biological Phenomenon," pp. 39–65.

29. Singer is a utilitarian, technically a "preference utilitarian," and this phrase, "the greatest happiness of the greatest number," is taken from John Stuart Mill (1806–1873), after Jeremy Bentham (1748–1832) the most prominent exponent of utilitarian ethics. In his *Utilitarianism* (various editions, see chapter two), Mill defines good as pleasure and the absence of pain, evil as pain and the absence of pleasure, and the "Greatest Happiness Principle" as the fundamental principle of morality.

30. Robert M. Veatch, "The Impending Collapse of the Whole-Brain Definition of Death," *Hastings Center Report*, vol. 23, no. 4, 1993, 18–24, reprinted in *Ethical Issues in Modern Medicine*, pp. 152–160.

31. Peter Singer, *Animal Liberation*, Revised edition (New York: Avon Books, 1990). See especially chapters two and three in which he discusses animal experimentation and factory farming, respectively. He quite rightly points out that it is wrong to subordinate animal lives to business values, so that cruelty is justified in order to increase profits. Though Singer also holds that business values are inimical to human values, I am not sure he can sustain this point on the basis of his ethical theory, a matter that I discuss in chapter five. But see his "Altruism and Commerce: A Defense of Titmuss Against Arrow," *Philosophy and Public Affairs* 2, 1973, pp. 312–320, and *Marx* (New York: Hill and Wang, 1980).

32. See *Animal Liberation*, pp. 80–94, and many other passages in Singer's books and articles. The moral evil of speciesism is a theme especially in *Practical Ethics*, Second Edition (Cambridge: Cambridge University Press, 1993), and in *Rethinking Life and Death*. Our society is "fundamentally speciesist," according to Singer, which makes it very difficult or impossible for us to see the myriad ways in which we favor human beings unjustly and correspondingly abuse the other animals.

33. See Dennis Normile, "Gene Expression Differs in Human and Chimp Brains: Greatly elevated levels of gene expression compared with chimpanzees and rhesus macaques shed light on how our brains developed," *Science*, 292, 6 April 2001, pp. 44–45.

34. Interestingly enough, and consistently with his views on this topic, Singer has recently argued that our revulsion against bestiality is irrational. Since we, too, are animals, interspecies sex "ceases to be an offense to our status and dignity as human beings." See Cathy Young, "No Heavy Petting," *Boston Globe*, 11 April 2001, p. A19. Young quotes Singer's article, "Heavy Petting," which recently appeared in the online magazine *Nerve*.

35. He gets this idea from Sidgwick, *The Methods of Ethics*, Seventh edition (London: Macmillan, 1907), pp. 420–421. See Singer, "Sidgwick and Reflective Equilibrium," *Monist* 58, 1974, p. 511.

36. See note 2.

37. See Franz Brentano, *The Origin of Our Knowledge of Right and Wrong*, trans. Chisholm and Schneewind (London: Routledge & Kegan Paul, 1969), p. 32. n.43.

38. See Plato, *Republic*, Book V.

39. See *How are We to Live? Ethics in an Age of Self-Interest* (Amherst, NY: Prometheus Books, 1995), as well as his other books and articles. To Singer's great credit he has brought these issues before the public in an accessible manner, and has not hid in the ivory tower with so many other twentieth century philosophers.

40. See Antonio Damasio, *Descartes' Error: Emotion, Reason, and the Human Brain* (New York: Avon Books, 1994). See also Daniel Goleman, *Emotional Intelligence* (New York: Bantam Books, 1995), pp. 27–29 and 52–54. Goleman credits Damasio with "the counter-intuitive position that feelings are typically *indispensable* for rational decisions" (Goleman's emphasis).

41. See note 25.

Chapter Two

The Source of Moral Value

Singer rejects the idea that there is an objective source of moral value partly because he thinks that science has shown the physical universe to be devoid of meaning and purpose. From this it would follow that any meaning and purpose discernible to us is a product of our own desires and preferences and not an objective fact about the world. As he puts it:

> If the universe has not been constructed in accordance with any plan, it has no meaning to be discovered. There is no value inherent in it, independently of the existence of sentient beings who prefer some states of affairs to others. Ethics is no part of the structure of the universe, in the way that atoms are.[1]

So in addition to rejecting traditional moral principles such as the sanctity of human life, as we saw in chapter one, Singer also rejects the worldview he takes those principles to be based on, namely the worldview according to which there is a Creator with a plan and hence an objectively discernible meaning of life. If moral value cannot be grounded in an objective reality that manifests the purposes of God, then it must be grounded subjectively in the preferences of the beings to whom moral value makes a difference.

SINGER'S CRITIQUE OF THE OBJECTIVITY OF MORAL VALUE

Singer's case against the objectivity of moral value is more sophisticated than it may at first appear, however. It is not just that he rejects the traditional theistic worldview, for that is only one way of establishing objective moral value. To be sure, if human beings were created by God in his image, then they would have intrinsic moral value by nature; but they might also be said to have intrinsic moral value on some other basis. The correctness of mathematics gives us an illustration. Even if there were no God and no plan or purpose behind the physical universe, it would still be true always and everywhere that 2+2=4. This would be an objective, necessary truth even if it were only a product of human thinking. The same would hold for the laws of logic such as the law of non-contradiction. That is to say, it is a mistake to contradict yourself, and even if humans are the only beings who perceive this, even if it is only a human truth, still its truth is objectively necessary in the sense that as far as we are concerned there can be no exceptions. So if it could be shown that reason itself somehow decrees that human beings have intrinsic moral value, then this value could be regarded as objectively grounded.

Singer agrees with the British philosopher, David Hume (1711–1776), however, that reason can perform no such function:

'Tis not contrary to reason to prefer the destruction of the whole world to the scratching of my finger. 'Tis not contrary to reason for me to choose my total ruin, to prevent the least uneasiness of an Indian or person wholly unknown to me. 'Tis as little contrary to reason to prefer even my own acknowledged lesser good to my greater, and have a more ardent affection for the former than the latter.[2]

In other words, there is no contradiction in preferring a lesser to a greater good. This is a very important point, crucial to understanding Singer on this issue. For if reason has nothing to say about preferring a lesser to a greater good, it follows that reason has nothing to say about preference at all.[3] A wedge is driven between rationality on the one hand and preference or desire on the other, such that absolutely any preference or desire could in principle count as not irrational. But if this is true, then reason as such has no decisive voice in ethics at the most fundamental level where moral value is discerned.

A couple of examples may make this clear. Consider ethical egoism, first of all. This is the position that whatever I want, because I perceive it to be to my advantage, is a morally legitimate object for me to pursue. As an egoist, I "look out for number one" and relegate the interests of others to second place at best.[4] Other persons are simply resources for my own projects, and to be treated as my advantage dictates. If Hume and Singer are right, this is not an irrational policy, though it may be an immoral one. There is no purely rational argument against egoism, because there is no contradiction in adopting it. What the egoist needs, from the ethical point of view, is a different set of preferences; but by hypothesis, this is precisely what the egoist lacks, and so long as the lack persists there is no rational argument that could provide a motive for reform.

Again, consider the psychopath[5] whose way of life is abhorrent to virtually everyone else, but who finds contentment in it nevertheless and sees no need to change. Relatives and friends may be desperate for a cure, but not the afflicted person. We may be tempted to say that "normal" people think clearly about human moral behavior and psychopaths do not; but in fact it is not a matter of clear thinking or rationality at all. Rather what is involved is a set of preferences that most people do not share, plus the inability to feel ordinary human emotions.

The egoist and the psychopath show us that reason is powerless to provide an objective source of moral value. The German philosopher, Immanuel Kant (1724–1804), had thought that ethics could be generated out of purely rational considerations. His so-called categorical imperative, "Act only according to that maxim by which you can at the same time will that it should become a universal law,"[6] was an attempt to place preference or desire under the direction of reason; but if Hume and Singer are right, the attempt was doomed to fail. For preference and desire function entirely independently of reason, and if anything, reason is under their direction. But preference and desire are subjective; and so the source of moral value is subjective and non-rational, according to Singer.

SINGER'S PROPOSAL THAT SUBJECTIVE PREFERENCE BE THE BASIS OF MORALITY

There being "no value inherent in [the universe], independently of the existence of sentient beings," it is the interests and preferences of sentient beings that constitute the whole source of moral value for Singer. In order to understand fully what Singer means by this, it is ultimately necessary to examine what he calls the "principle of the equal consideration of interests," but that is a topic to be saved for chapter four. Here we will examine how individual preference functions as the foundation of Singer's ethics; then in chapter three we will examine the role of reason in his ethics, given that (as we have just seen) it cannot have a foundational role. Having dealt with these two topics, we shall then be in a position to examine what Singer proposes as being the fundamental moral principle and its ramifications.

As noted earlier, Singer is a utilitarian, or more specifically, a preference utilitarian. Classical (or maximizing) utilitarianism seeks to maximize the amount of happiness in the world, meaning by 'happiness' pleasure and the absence of pain.[7] Preference utilitarianism, by contrast, seeks as much as possible to produce states of affairs that accord with the preferences of all who are affected by a given action or its consequences. The difference between the two versions of utilitarianism is roughly that classical utilitarianism is simpler; according to it, actions are good insofar as they promote the general happiness and bad insofar as they diminish the general happiness. Since happiness is defined as pleasure and the absence of pain, classical utilitarianism recommends the conceptually simple policy of maximizing pleasure and minimizing pain for the majority in the long run. Preference utilitarianism is more complex as a moral theory. It makes use of the concept of an individual's interest, which is understood to be what an individual prefers or, in the case of a rational agent, what an individual prefers "on balance and after reflection on all the relevant facts."[8] According to preference utilitarianism, then, actions are good insofar as they satisfy the interests of those affected and bad insofar as they fail to satisfy those interests. Thus preference utilitarianism recommends a policy somewhat more sophisticated than that promoted by classical utilitarianism, because preference utilitarianism makes use of the concepts of preference and interest in such a way that the satisfaction of interests may be understood to go beyond the simple maximization of pleasure and minimization of pain for the majority in the long run. At the same time, preference utilitarianism takes into account the interests of all sentient beings, just as classical utilitarianism takes into account their pleasure and pain; that is to say, neither version of utilitarianism restricts its sphere of application to rational beings, since simple sentience is all that is needed for an individual to feel pleasure or pain, or to have interests.[9]

Let us now take a look at two applications of Singer's preference utilitarianism. In his *Practical Ethics*, in the chapter entitled, "What's Wrong with Killing?" Singer tells us that preference utilitarianism defines as wrong any action that goes against the preference of any sentient being, except if the preference is outweighed by other contrary preferences. Thus killing a person whose preference is to continue living is wrong, all things equal. Moreover:

For preference utilitarians, taking the life of a person will normally be worse than taking the life of some other being, since persons are highly future-oriented in their preferences. . . . In contrast, beings who cannot see themselves as entities with a future cannot have any preferences about their own future existence.[10]

Of course, non-future-oriented beings may also struggle to escape or to live when threatened with pain or death, but this only means that they want the threatening situation to cease. Singer's preference utilitarianism provides guidelines for decision-making, then, that involve consideration of the interests of sentient beings in such a way that what the affected individuals subjectively prefer is indicative of right and wrong courses of action.

The first of the two applications I would like to consider involves the factors bearing on the decision to abort a pregnancy. What follows, however, is by no means a complete discussion of the topic of abortion, nor even of Singer's views on it. Rather, what I intend is simply to explore some aspects of the role of subjective preference in this area, in order to illuminate the role of subjective preference in Singer's ethics generally.

The interests involved in a decision to terminate pregnancy are typically those of the fetus and its parents. According to Singer, the interests of the fetus are like those of non-human animals who are incapable of conscious thought, namely, interests involving immediate pleasure and pain. The interests of the parents are normally more complex, that is to say they involve not only immediate pleasure and pain but also foreseeable pleasure and pain as well as any variety of future-oriented preferences and projects that adult human beings and perhaps some of the higher non-human animals may have. For Singer this means that the parents' interests are ordinarily decisive. For instance, if the fetus has some known abnormality that would cause it to live a life of severe and unremitting pain, then Singer says our usual intuitions tell us that it would be wrong to bring such a baby into the world. But otherwise, supposing its prospects for a fairly pleasant life are good, or at least not remarkably bad, even though the fetus itself has no awareness of a future, the parents are not wrong to want to bring the baby to term. But they are also not wrong to decide, should circumstances of whatever kind so move them, to terminate the pregnancy. This is because they are not wrong to put their own interests ahead of the fetus's interests, since they are conscious and aware of a future but the fetus is not.

This general position on the morality of abortion has the ramification (which Singer readily admits) of rendering infanticide also permissible in certain kinds of circumstance, namely, when the parents decide quite early in the infant's life[11] that they prefer not to raise the child. The case is no different from that of abortion, because the interests involved are weighted the same, the infant being capable of pleasure and pain but not self-aware and not oriented toward the future. Thus according to Singer it could be wrong to let the infant live if its life were foreseeably more painful than pleasant, and it is also permissible to kill the infant painlessly should the parents judge that to be in their interests. For the interests of the parents are decisive, within reason:

We should certainly put very strict conditions on permissible infanticide; but these restrictions might owe more to the effects of infanticide on others than to the intrinsic wrongness of killing an infant. Obviously, in most cases, to kill an infant is to inflict a terrible loss on those who love and cherish the child. . . . Thus infanticide can only be equated with abortion when those closest to the child do not want it to live. . . . Killing an infant whose parents do not want it dead is, of course, an utterly different matter.[12]

Singer's thinking on this topic is prompted partly by advances in modern medicine—we can now know ahead of time that an infant will be born with *spina bifida*, for instance—but also by the ages-old dilemma of what to do with an infant who has a condition such as Down's syndrome or something worse, which will make its life and the lives of others more or less difficult. As is obvious, based on our discussion in chapter one, Singer does not approach such a dilemma from the viewpoint of the sanctity of human life. Rather he agrees more with the ancient Greeks and Romans, who thought infanticide the humane solution in some cases.[13] But our concern here is primarily Singer's view of the source of moral value, and so the important point for our present purposes is that the rightness or wrongness of taking the life of a fetus or an infant is understood mainly in terms of the preferences and interests of the adults involved.[14]

Likewise, at the other end of life, Singer would decide the tough cases by weighing the interests of those affected. An elderly person who is sick and in pain, who freely decides not to go on living, should be able to opt for voluntary euthanasia. Again Singer's argument is an expression of preference utilitarianism:

Possibly the legalization of voluntary euthanasia would, over the years, mean the deaths of a few people who would otherwise have recovered from their immediate illness and lived for some extra years. This is not, however the knockdown argument against euthanasia that some imagine it to be. Against a very small number of unnecessary deaths that might occur if euthanasia is legalized we must place the very large amount of pain and distress that will be suffered if euthanasia is not legalized, by patients who really are terminally ill.[15]

For Singer, the decisive factor governing the question whether to kill someone who prefers not to go on living is precisely the person's desire not to go on living. This is evident because he takes it as obvious that in the aggregate the interests of a majority who wish to end their lives outweigh the interests of a minority who may be killed unnecessarily and/or against their will if voluntary euthanasia becomes legal.

Again, this is hardly a comprehensive account of Singer's views on euthanasia, but our purpose here is only to illustrate that the source of moral value for Singer is subjective preference. In sorting out the difficulties of the moral questions surrounding the issues of abortion, infanticide, and euthanasia, Singer repeatedly makes the fundamental appeal to subjective preference. It is both the starting point and the ultimate judge of the rightness or wrongness of an act. It is the source of ethics. It is even the criterion of the value of human existence.

Subjective preference is a more fundamental notion for Singer than is the concept of a right, for instance, the right to life. For all sentient beings have preferences in virtue of their capacity to feel pleasure and pain, but not all sentient beings are said to have rights. All sentient beings have interests, then, but not all sentient beings have interests that might be protected by the granting of rights to them. Only those sentient beings who are both rational and self-aware have interests that might be thus respected, for only they are persons, and only persons can be said to have rights.[16] Singer draws a line, that is, between animals that are merely sentient and animals that are persons. As we have seen, human fetuses and infants (up to perhaps a month of age) are not rational, self-aware and future-oriented, and so they do not qualify as persons. There are some non-human animals, however, that do appear to be rational, self-aware, and future-oriented and that do, therefore, qualify as persons. Thus for Singer the line between persons and non-persons does not coincide with the line (if it can be drawn)[17] between humans and non-humans.

Two crucial points emerge from this consideration of Singer's belief that subjective preference is the source of moral value. First of all, moral

value is fundamentally a subjective, psychological consideration grounded
in the preferences of individuals who can feel pleasure and pain. Secondly,
moral standing in the sense of having a right to life is also derived from a
subjective, psychological consideration, namely the capacity for rational, self-aware thought and the consciousness of oneself as persisting
through time (future-orientation).

PREFERENCE UTILITARIANISM AS A PRACTICAL ETHICAL THEORY

Singer's ethical theory, preference utilitarianism, is intended to be a
practical alternative to ethical theories that rely on supposedly objective
principles which people cannot agree about and which run into insur-
mountable difficulties of application in modern times. As such it has
three main features to recommend it: (1) it is subjectively grounded in a
way that any human being can accept; (2) it is not committed to any indefensible, absolute principles; (3) the interests of persons (of whatever
species) are guaranteed their rightful priority over the interests of sentient non-persons. Let us consider each of these features in turn.

First of all, the subjective grounding of Singer's ethics, its foundation
in subjective preference, takes into consideration the interests of any
sentient creature in such a way that there really is no requirement beyond sentience in order that the foundation be acceptable. There is no
need to commit to any religious creed or even any secular belief system,
since subjective preference is entirely pre-conceptual and understood,
as it were, by every sentient creature purely in terms of pleasure and
pain. This is something that sentient creatures can easily have in common with one another, something that binds us all together, rather
than being a divisive force that concepts and beliefs which fall short of
universal acceptance tend to be. Moreover, as Singer points out, since
preference utilitarianism takes the interests of *all* sentient beings into
account (i.e., since it universalizes) it takes the required step beyond
self-interest into ethics proper. Preference utilitarianism is thus a minimal ethics, and an adequate one. Therefore "the onus of proof [is] on
those who seek to go beyond utilitarianism."[18]

Secondly, though, if we were to go beyond preference utilitarianism
we would have to introduce further principles of some kind, and these
principles could only function in one of two ways: (1) they could be
relativized to individual preference; that is, subordinated to it and applied only insofar as they tended to produce states of affairs that satisfy a
majority of individual preferences; or else, (2) they could be absolutized

in such a way that individual preferences would be subordinated to the principles. The first option is equivalent to preference utilitarianism. But the second option is unacceptable because absolute moral principles are typically unworkable. Singer provides numerous examples of cases to which the ethical principles that would go beyond utilitarianism simply do not apply.[19] To cite just three kinds of situations that he has in mind, consider (1) a brain-dead woman who turns out to be pregnant, or (2) an anencephalic infant whose organs would benefit an infant who has a complete brain, or (3) the thousands of people who live on in a persistent vegetative state.[20] By applying the ethics of preference utilitarianism we can deal with these cases for we can easily know the factors that should apply. Neither the brain-dead woman nor her fetus has interests (except insofar as the fetus may be able to feel pain) and so the preferences and interests of their family and close friends should be decisive. The anencephalic infant has no interests but the infant who could benefit from its organs does, and so do the respective families, whose wishes should be respected and mediated for the benefit of the greater number should a dispute arise. The thousands of people in vegetative states are individuals who have no interests, except perhaps to the extent that they are able to feel pain; again, the preferences of their loved ones are decisive. In every such case, provided no needless pain is inflicted, preference utilitarianism is adaptable to the wishes of the majority of conscious, future-oriented individuals involved.

By contrast, ethical systems that impose principles beyond the utilitarian lead inevitably to unresolvable dilemmas. Suppose for instance that we take it as always wrong to bring about the death of an innocent human being. At a minimum, application of this principle in the cases mentioned will mean severe hardship for the conscious and rational individuals involved. Though there is nothing hard and fast about this in Singer's view, and the family's preference may be to raise an infant whose mother is brain-dead or to keep a loved one alive in a persistent vegetative state indefinitely, still those (perhaps a majority) who would reject these prospects are not morally in the wrong and should not be made to feel so. Moreover in the second case, that of the anencephalic infant, our adherence to the absolute principle will actually mean that we cannot escape violating the principle itself. For if we decide to maintain the life of the anencephalic infant, then we must sacrifice the life of the infant who could be saved by its organs, and conversely, if we save the life of the infant who has a complete brain we must sacrifice the life of the anencephalic infant.[21] According to Singer, it would have to be proved that the further principle was beneficial, but in fact it appears to be harmful instead. Not only that, but the principle's ultimate break-down under pressure shows that our traditional morality is rotten in its foundations, or as he says it, "crumbling at the edges."[22] Therefore Singer's preference utilitarianism, with its basis in subjective prefer-ence, is better than any theory that would commit us to indefensible ab-solute moral principles.

Thirdly, because of the way the terms 'preference' and 'interest' are understood, preference utilitarianism naturally guarantees the priority of the interests of conscious, rational, and future-oriented beings over the interests of those that are merely sentient. This is an advantage of the theory because it agrees with our intuitions in various kinds of cases. Singer repeatedly appeals to common moral judgments of our day in re-gard to such issues as abortion and euthanasia. Because a majority agree that abortion within some shorter or longer period of gestation is per-missible subject to the preferences of the mother (and perhaps to a lesser extent the father), therefore we should recognize a similar per-missibility of infanticide within certain parameters. Because a majority agree that "passive" euthanasia ("pulling the plug," for instance) is per-missible when an elderly patient desires no further treatment, therefore we should recognize a similar permissibility of "active" euthanasia (as-sisted suicide or lethal injection) within certain parameters. Consis-tency in application of the subjective preference criterion, and respect for the subjective determination of the value of a life—the value to oth-ers in the case of non-persons, and the value to the person herself or himself in other cases[23]—will lead to a morally clarified, humane soci-ety, according to Singer.

REPLY TO SINGER ON OBJECTIVITY

Given that "ethics is no part of the structure of the universe," as Singer says, does it follow that the basis of ethics cannot be objective in any meaningful sense? We have seen already that if ethics were founded somehow in rationality then it could be said to have an objective foun-dation. As has been pointed out by Hume and others, however, there are problems with adopting that view. Singer ultimately concludes that at best the only element of objectivity in the foundation of ethics that reason can provide is the universal perspective according to which oth-ers' interests count as much as my own do in my moral decision making. We shall examine this claim in chapter three. For the moment let us take a closer look at Singer's critique of the objectivity of moral value.

Though he does not claim that the only way to have a coherent view of objective moral value is to believe in a Creator with a plan for humanity, nevertheless there is a sense in which Singer's whole ethical outlook is premised on the falsehood of traditional religion. In fact, however, there is no need for ethics to have a religious basis in order for it to include belief in objective moral value. In ancient times, Platonists, Aristotelians, and Stoics all regarded moral value as having a basis in human nature, and they regarded human nature as an objective reality. It is true that the existence of human nature has been called into question, especially in the twentieth century, and certainly Singer rejects it based on what we discussed in chapter one concerning the definition of the human species. Singer also tends to see belief in the existence of a human nature as tied to theism. Still, it is possible to see ethical behavior as Aristotle did—as the normative, healthy functioning of a biological organism on the earth, in other words, as an objective reality. And it is possible to see ethics as Plato and the Stoics did—as the exemplification in human affairs of the eternal and universal moral law, the idea of justice, again an objective reality. Why does Singer insist otherwise?

Ultimately it is Singer's view of reason that is decisive here. When Hume pointed out that reason cannot be the basis of ethics he understood 'reason' in a specific way, and Singer follows him in this, as do perhaps the majority of philosophers since the time of Hume with the exception of Kant and his followers. Without engaging the technicalities of this debate in modern philosophy, suffice it to say that 'reason' may be understood broadly in two ways:[24] (1) it may be understood as a calculative faculty, a logical activity, which determines what follows from what; or (2) it may be understood as a faculty of insight, an intuitive or insightful activity, which discerns the essence or nature of a thing. It is in the first sense that Hume and Singer understand reason, and this is why they say it cannot generate ethics or determine moral value. When they tell us there is nothing irrational in preferring a lesser to a greater good, then, they are absolutely right, but they only mean that from the fact that I prefer a lesser to a greater good it does not follow by the rules of logic that I am mistaken in doing so. " 'Tis not contrary to reason," as Hume puts it. But suppose we use the term 'reason' in the second sense noted above and apply it to a preference that will strike most people as quite strange. Apparently there are a group of gay men who have founded a kind of subculture on the basis of preferring to transmit and receive HIV.[25] They call their initiates "bugchasers" and imagine themselves as the "fathers" of those they infect, and as the "sons" of those by whom they have been infected, thus constituting an aberrant "family." 'Tis not contrary to reason, in the first sense above; there is no contradiction in their preferring to contract AIDS rather than not contracting it. But it is indeed contrary to reason in the second sense above, because it involves a completely mistaken intuition or insight about family, community, and the nature and value of human life.

Admittedly, my second sense of 'reason' would not be acceptable usage to Hume or to Singer, because they would reject the idea that the human intellect possesses such a power. Though philosophical tradition would be on my side, the majority opinion in recent decades would probably be on their side. It doesn't matter. The point is only that you do not do away with objectivity in the foundation of ethics by claiming that there is no God and that no subjective preferences are irrational. Certain preferences are beyond the pale for everybody—not the same ones, necessarily, for each of us, but all of us have limits as to what we can countenance as being morally right. Singer is no exception, as we can see when we read what he has to say about eating the "bodies of animals."[26] So all of us, whether we like it or not, must *assume* that there is an element of objectivity in the foundation of ethics.[27] For instance in the example of the "bugchasers" above, either you agree with my assessment or you disagree with it. In either case, you employ your faculty of rational intuition or insight and make an objective judgment—to the effect that the "bugchasers" are just fine doing whatever they want, or to the effect that they are confused about what is good for them. It is only at the rarefied level where we define the uses of 'reason' that it appears legitimate to reject reason's intuitive function. But even if it is true that reason has no such function, we are forced when we consider specific cases to behave *as if* it does. Therefore Singer is wrong to exclude objectivity from the foundation of ethics.

REPLY TO SINGER ON SUBJECTIVITY

But isn't Singer right to notice that when our supposedly rational intuition rejects something as obviously immoral what's really happening is that our subjective preferences are kicking in and, as Hume would put it, reason is the slave of the passions after all? No doubt this is exactly what happens in many instances. But for it to be true across the board, with no exceptions, something else would have to be true, namely, that nothing we apprehend subjectively is ever an objective truth. But this is demonstrably false.

The French philosopher, René Descartes (1596–1650), was perhaps the first to notice that a subjective insight can yield an objective truth.[28]

In reflecting on the unreliability of sense perception and traditional authority as sources of knowledge, he came to realize that even if he doubted everything he had ever learned he could still be certain of his own existence whenever he thought about anything at all. Thus his famous observation, "I think, therefore I am." The importance of Descartes' philosophy to developments in philosophy since his time, and in fact to the whole of modern culture, is incalculable in a wide variety of areas.[29] But we are focussing on just a tiny fraction of that influence here; he showed us that what an individual thinks privately and subjectively can have application and legitimacy publicly and objectively. Modern respect for the independence of an individual thinking person, where it exists and by sharp contrast with the individual's subordination to authority and received opinion, is a positive result of the Cartesian philosophy.[30] Granted we all have plenty of personal opinions that are mistaken, unwarranted, insupportable, or otherwise worthless. It remains true that our own existence, integrity, and some of our inner states are known to us with a certainty that cannot be impugned from the outside and that cannot be disparaged as merely subjective. The subjective is not necessarily non-objective. What is subjectively known may be true objectively, just as what is subjectively believed may be false objectively.

Subjective preference, as distinct from belief, is also capable of being correct or incorrect.[31] Again, the fact that something is subjectively discerned says nothing about whether it is objectively respectable; that is a separate consideration. When I say, "I think, therefore I am," I am on solid ground; when I say, "I know of no hazards in the area, therefore there are none," I am out on a limb. But in both cases the objective truth or falsehood of my statement is a function, not of subjective origin, but of verifiable fact. By analogy, if I say, "I feel that human life is intrinsically valuable, therefore humans should not kill one another," I may be on solid ground; but if I say, "I feel the 'bugchasers' are entitled to their lifestyle, therefore what they do is morally acceptable," I may be out on a limb, perhaps way out. Here the correctness or incorrectness of subjective preference is a function, not of subjective origin, but of human moral life. Let us grant to Singer, in other words, that we cannot do ethics or think morally without involving our subjective preferences and feelings at a fundamental level. It does not follow that the foundation of ethics is merely subjective, or subjective in a pejorative sense.

It may be, in fact, that like Descartes' "I think, therefore I am," the foundation of morality *has to be* subjectively perceived. It is possible, in other words, that the basis of ethics is our concern for human beings, because they are human. The value we place on human life, as a conse-

quence of our concern for humanity, is admittedly a subjective preference, then, but not one that is merely subjective in the sense that it
might not be objectively valid. So I suggest that though Singer may be
right to insist that subjective preference is the foundation of morality,
he is wrong to insist that there is no correctness or incorrectness of subjective preferences. Let us see what sort of change this would make to
the cases examined above in our discussion of preference utilitarianism.

Considering abortion, first of all, and again without giving the topic
a thorough treatment, let us ask whether the subjective preferences of
the persons involved really yield an ethically sound appraisal. Is it possible for a parent correctly to prefer the death of her or his fetus to its continued life? Notice that our question is not whether it is *possible* to prefer
the death of the fetus, but whether such a preference could possibly be
morally correct. How can we answer such a question? Will the answer
not depend on the circumstances? Suppose the fetus is unwanted, or
deformed, or doomed to a life of poverty and despair; in such cases
would it not be better off dead? Setting aside questions about whether
non-existent entities can have properties like being better off, the task
here is to think morally, not factually.[32] The facts may be whatever they
may be—rejection, deformity, poverty—but the moral question, the
question not about *what is* but about *what ought to be*, is different.
Ought a parent to prefer her or his fetus's death? Clearly not. It is unnat-
ural and wrong. To deny this is to deny our very human feeling that the
decision to abort a pregnancy is and should be an agonizing decision.

If our feeling to this effect has been dulled over recent decades, perhaps we can still evoke it by considering the case of infanticide. Just as a
fetus may be unwanted, deformed, or unable to be fed, so may an infant, and throughout history human beings have often felt forced by
circumstances to kill their own children. Is this not tragic? And must it
not have been an agonizing choice for the parents? Would it help if an
expert in ethics were to show conclusively that the preferences of the
parents are decisive?[33] Or if that could be shown, would we remain able
to distinguish between cruel parents who murder their children (to satisfy a preference) and desperate, wretched parents who could not feed
another mouth?

One problem with Singer's preference utilitarianism is that it tends
to erase the difference between a wanton act and a legitimate option.
This is partly because it lacks the distinction between correct and incorrect preference. But at the root of this is another problem, namely, the
absence of a truly human standard of right and wrong. How human beings *do* feel about one another, and how they *ought to* feel for one an-

other, are legitimate, foundational considerations in ethics which we ignore at our peril.

Consider again the case of euthanasia. Singer is right that it is entirely possible for an elderly person who is sick and in pain, with no hope of recovery, to prefer to die. He may even be right to hold that the person's family and friends should respect his or her wishes. But to prefer to die, and especially to prefer that our loved ones should die, is just wrong. Otherwise why would it be such a sad thing to come to this point?

Of course, Singer knows that we prefer life to death, other things equal, and that parents prefer that their children live and thrive, other things equal. He knows that our preferences concerning life are important, but he does not see them as anchored in the value of human life. Rather, reversing the priority, he sees the value of human life as a function of subjective preference. Thus, for Singer, the life of an infant or of a brain-dead adult has value only in terms of the preferences of family and close friends, and the life of an elderly person who is sick and in pain but conscious has value mainly in terms of the elderly person's preferences. To make his theory work he assumes, as we have seen, that subjective preferences are neither rational nor irrational as such and neither correct nor incorrect. So I think Singer's theory is wrong on two counts: (1) it is not true that subjective preferences are neither correct nor incorrect; and (2) human life does have intrinsic value grounded in an obviously correct subjective preference which in turn essentially determines the correctness (or incorrectness) of other subjective preferences. Granted, it may only be in some of the less extreme cases that this is crystal clear. If we prefer the death to the life of an elderly patient who is a pain in the neck to us and not mentally competent, we should pause and reflect on the intrinsic value of human life. If, on the other hand, a mother wonders whether to abort an anencephalic fetus, that is a tougher case. But behind it all there should be a sense that human life is precious, and that therefore we *should* agonize over the tough cases. Does this mean that we will be committed to indefensible absolute principles? Perhaps. At a minimum, it means that we will sometimes find ourselves in concrete situations where no matter what we do we shall not be able to rest easy with the confidence of having done the right thing.

REPLY TO SINGER ON PRACTICALITY

According to Singer and many others, however, it is possible to have ethics without the anguish.[34] It is thought to be possible on the basis of subjective preference, and a calculation of the effects on the aggregate of interests, to arrive at a clear sense of the right thing to do in every case. This is how Singer solves questions of life and death—abortion, infanticide, voluntary euthanasia, assisted suicide—and it is on this basis that he proposes a reform of ethics for our time, including a revision of the "moral commandments."[35]

In my opinion, however, it is neither possible nor even desirable to defuse the anguish of moral decision-making. Let us consider the possibility first.

Singer has introduced the subjective source of moral value as a device for cutting through fundamental disagreement about ethical principles that he sees as characterizing our society in an era of secularism and modern medicine. Beginning as utilitarians do with something we can all agree about, namely, that pleasure is preferable to pain, Singer proceeds to structure an ethics of theoretical plausibility and practical applicability that should arm us to face the difficult choices ahead as these are epitomized by dilemmas resulting from biomedical advances in our day. Just as the Harvard Committee sought to redefine death in order to facilitate the harvesting of organs for transplant, so Singer seeks to refashion ethics in order to defuse the agony we feel over pulling the plug on a loved one, aborting a deformed fetus, deciding not to feed a Down's syndrome infant, and "dying with dignity" when our own time comes. But is it humanly possible for us to face these kinds of decisions without anguish?

The mere fact that I prefer one state of affairs to another tells me nothing about whether I am right to do so. Suppose I prefer not to see an aged relative kept alive on machines, or suppose I prefer not to raise a Down's syndrome infant, the question then becomes, not whether I shall be able to satisfy my preferences, but rather, what is the right thing to do? For Singer, to be sure, the answer to this question is arrived at by taking into account the preferences and interests of *everyone* who will be affected, the idea being that if all are consulted the result will be a moral conclusion rather than a merely self-interested one. But it is not clear why the aggregate of preferences should be more enlightening about the right thing to do than an individual preference would be. The fact is, what is right is often precisely what we do *not* prefer, hence the pain of moral choice. Sometimes what is right coincides with what we prefer, sometimes it does not, and the task is to figure out in each case how the two are related and how to proceed from there.

The subjective preferences having been established, Singer would proceed by means of a calculus in which the interests of all are placed in a balance. There are ways of figuring out whose interests count for more, ways of being sure that interests are weighed fairly, and as we have seen, a priority given always to the interests of those who are persons (conscious, rational, and future-oriented). Even with the utmost faith in this system, however, and given the ideal case where a clear majority of interests can be satisfied, what assures me that I have arrived at a morally right conclusion as distinct from merely the correct calculation of relevant factors? It is in the deciding, and in hoping that one has decided rightly, that the moral life is lived. Even the result of a flawless calculation of relevant interests is open to the questioning of a moral agent. Suppose everyone agrees that we should disconnect the machines, or discontinue food and fluids—still I, if I face the decision, must make the decision in the hope that I do right.

Granted that some moral anguish is needless (being due either to ignorance or to excessive guilt), still neither subjective preference at the foundation nor careful calculation based on it can deliver us from all the difficulties—sometimes, the agonies—of deciding on a moral course of action. But even if we could be thus delivered, should we wish to be?

A large part of what it means to be human is our autonomy as moral agents. Part of what our autonomy involves is that, although we formulate and agree to the basic moral rules, we also individually decide where and how they should apply. This is true whether you think of morality as a God-given code or a man-made one. In either case there is our assent to the code, on the one hand, and our personal application of it on the other. Suppose this were taken away. That is, suppose the moral code decreed for every case exactly what ought to be done and the individual agent had only to apply the code to the case at hand. We would be living under a moral totalitarianism, either secular or religious. Singer's preference utilitarianism comes perilously close to the secular variety of moral totalitarianism in that it tends to obviate any need for an autonomous agent. Why would I question anymore the permissibility of refusing to feed a Down's syndrome infant, when the moral code tells me to do precisely as the properly weighted interests of the majority of those affected dictate? Why would I continue to bear responsibility including praise and blame for my decisions and subsequent actions, if the code itself had predetermined what they should be?

Lest we lose sight of the fact, it bears repeating that Singer's utilitarian calculus dictates what is right and wrong precisely in order to escape the unreasonable dictates of traditional morality. As we saw in chapter one, Singer finds traditional belief in the sanctity of human life, for instance, to be oppressive and limiting to us in the modern world of advanced medical technology. What he sets up in reaction against the tradition is a moral code which decrees, among other things, that it is morally acceptable to kill innocent human beings under certain kinds of circumstances. I do not wish to impute any kind of inhumane motive to Singer in this; far from it, his whole goal is to make ethics more adaptable to difficult human circumstances. But in this effort he runs the grave risk of losing the very thing that has always made ethics especially human and especially valuable to human civilization, that is, its provision of a transcendent standard of conduct that everybody knows we will at times fail to live up to.[36] It is no criticism of an ethical system that it is very hard to live up to, however. Rather, that is the whole idea! The normative differs from the factual, as we saw in chapter one, precisely in this, that *what is the case* is not always, and not necessarily, *what ought to be!* So morality itself *cannot* declare that sometimes it is morally permissible to kill an innocent human being.[37] Alas, we who may unhappily find ourselves guilty of innocent blood must bear the burden of it and admit what we have done. To fall short in this is not only moral cowardice—it is the demise of ethics. To explain away the taking of innocent human life in terms of the interests of parents, or family, or potential organ recipients, is a perversion of both reason and morality.

Nevertheless, it may be objected, the demands of real life situations can bring us to the point where the only reasonable course of action—perhaps taking the organs from a life we are sure to lose, in order to support a life we might thereby save—and the only practical solution to an agonizing state of affairs may be to opt out of traditional morality. The mindless application of principle without regard for the exigencies of real situations seems itself to be irrational, no matter how solid the arguments in favor of a given principle might be. This raises the question of reason's role in ethics generally, and in moral decision making in particular. We have seen that 'reason' is a term used with a variety of meanings, two of which we distinguished above, the sense of calculation and the sense of insight. Though Singer accepts the former, and rejects the latter, though he denies reason a role in ethics at the most fundamental level where moral value is discerned, yet there is an element of rational insight in his ethics, specifically at the level of the universalization of preferences. To this topic we turn in chapter three.

NOTES

1. Singer, *How Are We to Live? Ethics in an Age of Self-Interest* (New York: Prometheus Books, 1995), p. 188.

2. Singer, *Practical Ethics*, Second Edition (Cambridge: Cambridge University Press, 1993), p. 320. Hume's words are taken from *A Treatise of Human Nature*, bk. 2, pt. iii, sec. 3, which is also the source for his famous claim, "Reason is, and ought only to be the slave of the passions, and can never pretend to any other office than to serve and obey them." Singer is Humean on this point.

3. For a recent discussion of this topic see Dale Jamieson, ed., *Singer and His Critics* (Oxford: Blackwell, 1999), pp. 269–270, and 280–286.

4. For a "strongest case" analysis of amoral personal egoism, see John van Ingen, *Why Be Moral?* (New York: Peter Lang, 1994).

5. Singer uses this definition of a psychopath: "a person who is asocial, impulsive, egocentric, unemotional, lacking in feelings of remorse, shame, or guilt, and apparently unable to form deep and enduring personal relationships." See *Practical Ethics*, pp. 328–330.

6. Immanuel Kant, *Foundations of the Metaphysics of Morals*, trans. Lewis White Beck (Indianapolis: Bobbs-Merrill, 1959) [1785], Second Section, p. 39 [422].

7. The literature on utilitarianism generally, and on the special varieties of utilitarianism, is enormous. The classic source is John Stuart Mill's *Utilitarianism* (various editions). Singer's discussions may be found in *Practical Ethics*, especially chapter one, and in several articles, notably: "Is Act Utilitarianism Self-Defeating?" *Philosophical Review* 81, 1972, pp. 94–104; and "Possible Preferences," in Christoph Fehige and Ulla Wessels, eds., *Preferences* (Berlin and New York: Walter deGruyter, 1998), pp. 383–398.

8. Singer, *Practical Ethics*, p. 94. Any sentient being may be said to have preferences and interests, as these terms are understood here. For Singer, a 'person' is a rational and self-aware being. (See *Practical Ethics*, p. 87.) The interests of sentient beings who are persons sometimes carry more moral weight, so to speak, than the interests of sentient beings who are not persons. For Singer, some human beings are not persons, and some non-human animals are persons. (See, among other sources, *Practical Ethics*, pp. 83–89.)

9. This is just one way to look at the comparison, however. A different conceptual analysis may find classical utilitarianism more complex and preference utilitarianism simpler. There is something to be said for this account, since, for instance, Mill's utilitarianism with "higher" and "lower" pleasures introduces considerations that Singer's preference utilitarianism seems to do without. Mill's utilitarianism likewise seems to me more humane than Singer's. See Mill, *Utilitarianism*, especially chapter two, where he writes, "It is better to be a human being dissatisfied than a pig satisfied; better to be Socrates dissatisfied than a fool satisfied. And if the fool, or the pig, are of a different opinion, it is because they only know their own side of the question. The other party to the comparison knows both sides."

10. *Practical Ethics*, pp. 94–95.

11. Singer has proposed time periods of twenty-eight days, or a month, but has conceded that the exact window of permissibility is a matter for some disagreement, medically speaking. The crucial consideration, of course, is whether the infant is not merely aware of pain and pleasure but also conscious in the sense of being conscious of its own existence in time and able to feel fear and to anticipate pain. See Singer, *Rethinking Life and Death: The Collapse of Our Traditional Ethics* (New York: St. Martin's Press, 1994), pp. 180–183 and 210–219.

12. Singer, *Practical Ethics*, pp. 173–174. This is the conclusion of chapter six, "Taking Life: The Embryo and the Fetus," which begins p. 135.

13. He cites Plato, Aristotle, and Seneca (see *Practical Ethics*, p. 173), praising Seneca especially for his compassion. None of these thinkers, however, believed that the source of moral value is subjective; rather they found it objectively, in the nature of things.

14. For Singer, the permissibility of both abortion and infanticide presupposes that care will be taken not to inflict pain on the fetus or infant. Painful methods of abortion or infanticide are to be avoided. See *Practical Ethics*, pp. 164–165, where Singer suggests that somewhere between eighteen and thirty weeks' gestation the fetus begins to be capable of being harmed (in the sense that non-self-aware but sentient non-humans can be) and of feeling pain.

15. See Singer, *Practical Ethics*, pp. 196–197, and *Rethinking Life and Death*, p. 146. Singer places great faith in the guidelines of the Royal Dutch Medical Association, which require among other things that death be explicitly requested by the patient, who is well-informed of any alternatives for alleviating suffering, and that euthanasia must be carried out by a physician who has consulted with a second, independent medical professional. Singer claims that there is no evidence that the rate of murder has increased in the Netherlands since euthanasia has been legal there; presumably only the rate of killing has gone up.

16. See *Practical Ethics*, p. 87, and *Rethinking Life and Death*, pp. 180–183.

17. Notice that the more objective line, between one species and another, seems to be less discernible to Singer than the more subjective line, between the conscious and the non-conscious, or the future-oriented and the non-future-oriented.

18. *Practical Ethics*, p. 14. It would have to be proved, in other words, that ethics actually requires more than what preference utilitarianism provides. I believe that ethics does require more.

19. See especially *Rethinking Life and Death*, chapters one through seven.

20. Estimates of the number of patients in persistent vegetative state in the United States in 1992 range from 14,000 to 35,000. See *Rethinking Life and Death*, p. 59.

21. Singer rejects the usual distinction between acts and omissions in favor of emphasis on the end result. See *Rethinking Life and Death*, pp. 75–80.

22. See *Rethinking Life and Death*, p. 81.

23. Note that not only are some human beings not persons, for Singer, while some non-human beings are persons, but also a given individual can go from being a person to being a non-person, too, since personhood is defined in terms of a set of properties that an individual can acquire and lose over time.

24. See, for instance, Heidegger, "Memorial Address on the 175th Birthday of Conradin Kreutzer," in his *Discourse on Thinking* (New York: Harper & Row, 1966), translation of *Gelassenheit* by John M. Anderson and E. Hans Freund, pp. 43–57. See also Thomas Aquinas on the distinction between *scientia* and *intellectus*, in *Summa Theologiae*, II a, q. 57, a2.

25. See *Boston Globe*, 18 June 2000, p. A18.

26. See *Animal Liberation*, p. 214.

27. This does not prove that there is such an objective element, of course; it only says that we will always be stymied if we try to prove there is no such element, because we will be assuming there is. Consider what happens when moral relativists object to moral absolutists on the grounds that moral absolutism leads to immoral consequences; the relativists have made an absolutist claim. Nor is it mere logical trickery to point this out; rather it tells us something important about moral discourse, namely, that qua normative it is objectivist.

28. See Descartes, *Meditations on First Philosophy*, various editions, Meditations One and Two. Arguably St. Augustine anticipated this, however, when he pointed out that "if I err, I exist." See *On Free Choice of the Will*, various editions, Book Two, chapter three.

29. Descartes' dualism is his most famous contribution, and certainly has had a huge effect on modern culture. The ease with which we imagine ourselves occupied by or inhabiting the bodies of "space aliens," and our capacity to entertain the prospect of our "identity" being saved in digital form on a computer after our death speak volumes about this. But I am focussing far more narrowly here, our Cartesian culture in the West being the topic for a separate book.

30. Other positive results are to be found in nineteenth and early twentieth century psychology, for instance in the work of Franz Brentano and Edmund Husserl, as well as Freud and others. See, among other sources, Brentano, *Psychology From an Empirical Standpoint*, trans. Rancurello, Terrell, and McAlister (New York: Humanities Press, 1973).

31. Among those who have emphasized this point, Franz Brentano especially deserves mention. See *The Origin of Our Knowledge of Right and Wrong*, trans. Chisholm and Schneewind (London: Routledge and Kegan Paul, 1969).

32. Philosophers do discuss such questions. See Derek Parfit, *Reasons and Persons* (Oxford: Clarendon Press, 1984), Appendix G, "Whether Causing Someone to Exist Can Benefit This Person," pp. 487–490.

33. In arguing against Singer's utilitarianism and in favor of an "ethic of reciprocity," Nel Noddings notes: "an ethic of caring strives consistently to capture our human intuitions and feelings. We cannot accept an ethic that depends upon a definition of personhood if that definition diminishes our obligation to human infants. An ethic that forces us to classify human infants with rats and pigs is unsettling [sic]. We feel intuitively that something must be wrong with it." See her *Caring: A Feminine Approach to Ethics and Moral Education* (Berkeley and Los Angeles: University of California Press, 1984), p. 151. See also Singer, Kuhse, and Rickard, "Reconciling Impartiality and a Feminist Ethic of Care," *Journal of Value Inquiry*, 32 (1998), pp. 451–463.

34. See especially, R.M. Hare, *Moral Thinking: Its Levels, Method and Point* (Oxford: Clarendon Press, 1981), p. 26. Hare's famous distinction between the intuitive level and the critical level in moral thinking plays a key role in Singer's moral philosophy. Hare claims that the view that there really are irresolvable moral conflicts is due to a failure to distinguish the intuitive level (where the conflicts appear) from the critical level (where the conflicts disappear). It does seem to be true that moral principles themselves should not be in conflict, i.e., that the conflicts arise in application. But since we live in the real world, and not in the world of theory, we can all expect to face situations where the conflict of duty leads to anguish. It is one thing to realize that we *have to* decide, in such cases; it is another to claim, after the fact, that there really had been a correct solution all along. The latter is what I doubt.

35. See *Rethinking Life and Death*, Chapter Nine, "In Place of the Old Ethic," especially pp. 190–206.

36. To a certain extent, Singer makes up for this in his work on animal liberation and on the obligations of the affluent to the needy, but then this is accomplished by shifting the ground of moral anxiety from human to non-human affairs, and from the concerns of those close to us to the concerns of those at a further remove. The general revised picture of the moral life emerges best in Singer, *How Are We To Live?*

37. Again, Nel Noddings is eloquent on the point: "Locating our primary obligation in the domain of human life is a logical outgrowth of the fact that ethicality is defined in the human domain—that the moral attitude would not exist or be recognized without human affection and rational reflection upon or assessment of that affection. It is not 'speciesism' to respond differently to different species if the very form of response is species specific." See *Caring*, p. 152. The source of moral value is located in our regard for one another as human, and if this be speciesism or mindless adherence to inbred preferences, then that is what ethics turns out to be.

Chapter Three

The Role of Reason in Ethics

In addition to the senses of the term 'reason' as calculation and as insight, noted in chapter two, we might also distinguish the sense of reason as an aid in acquiring factual knowledge about the world. We might say, for instance, that medical researchers *reasoned* their way through to the cause of malaria or of bubonic plague. This kind of reasoning is causal or experimental. It differs from what I have called calculative reasoning in that it is about events in the world, not about logic or mathematics, and it differs from insight in that it is about what happens rather than what is; i.e., it is about events or occurrences, not about the categories or values of things. Though I have now distinguished three senses of the term, 'reason,' because it will clarify certain points I want to make about Singer's arguments, I make no claim that this is an adequate analysis of the concept.[1] Perhaps further senses of the term, 'reason,' could be usefully distinguished. Nor do I intend to impute my distinctions to Singer. He does make a general claim about reason—that it has non-foundational uses in ethics, e.g., in discerning relevant facts, and in promoting the universal point of view, though not in governing preferences—but he does not distinguish senses of the term. So

the distinctions are part of my program, not his, and again the senses of
the term 'reason' are three: let us call them calculative reason, intuitive
reason, and experimental reason.

In this chapter, we will take up two main topics concerning the role
of reason in ethics. The first is its fact finding role, the job of what I call
experimental reason. We shall examine two instances presented by
Singer in which a correct assessment of the facts makes a difference, he
says, in the moral analysis of cases. The first instance we have not discussed earlier, namely, recent biological findings about the so-called
"moment of conception" of a human embryo. The second instance we
have looked at already briefly in chapter one, namely, recent findings
about the genetic relationship between humans and chimpanzees.

The second role of reason to be examined is its universalizing role, a
task of what I call intuitive reason. According to Singer, the distinctly
moral question, "What if everybody did that?" involves each of us in the
realization that the interests of every sentient creature are equally as important as our own, so that eventually rational reflection leads us to the
insight he calls the "principle of equal consideration of interests." The
principle itself will be examined in chapter four, but the mode of arriv-
ing at it will be the topic of the second half of this chapter.

SINGER ON "EXPERIMENTAL" REASON AS AN
AID TO ETHICAL THINKING

In chapter three of his *Rethinking Life and Death*, "Uncertain Beginnings," in the sections entitled, "New Reproductive Technology
and the Abortion Debate," and "Unlocking the Abortion Deadlock,"
Singer explores the so-called "moment of conception" as an alleged
fact employed in arguments against abortion. Such arguments typically
reason that because it is wrong to take innocent human life, and because the embryo or fetus is human from conception onwards, therefore it is wrong to take the life of the embryo or fetus.[2] But as Singer
points out, it is not at all clear either (1) that there is a *moment* of conception or (2) that in its early stages the embryo is a human *individual*.[3]

First, it is not clear that there is a *moment* of conception, according to
Singer, because the coming into being of a human individual is a grad-
ual process rather than an instantaneous occurrence. It may be thought
that the joining together of the sperm and the egg constitutes a beginning point for the individual (or, as we shall see, individual*s*) who
uniquely bears the resulting DNA "fingerprint." But in fact the genetic
materials from the sperm and from the egg are not joined until some

time later, in a process known as "syngamy," which occurs in the nucleus of the single cell they gradually form. Science has thus shown us that, in place of a mysterious first moment of existence, human beings have in their early stages a step-by-step career no moment of which can be singled out as the moment before which there is no new human being and after which there is one.

Secondly, according to Singer, it is not clear that even starting at the point of syngamy what exists is a single human *individual.* The possibility of twinning persists for some days after the zygote is fully formed; but if the zygote is potentially two (or more) individuals, then it is not true to say of it that it constitutes one, unique human being. Again, the light shed by science allows us to see the origin of human individuals, not as an abrupt occurrence, but as a natural process over time in which the status of the entity involved necessarily cannot be clearly pinpointed at any given moment. Beyond a certain stage, twinning is no longer a possibility, and then it is safe to say that we are dealing with a specific number of human individuals based on the constitution of the embryo or embryos. Though no exact moment can be designated, apparently it is safe to say that after fourteen days beyond syngamy, the resulting human beings could in principle be counted.

The biological evidence about individuality and about the alleged "moment of conception" has ramifications for ethics, according to Singer. This is reason in its experimental use being applied to aid decision-making in the normative realm. For once we realize that a zygote is no more to be thought of as a human individual than its predecessor sperm or egg were, then we can apply this knowledge to questions, for example, about how to deal with the extra zygotes that result from attempts at *in vitro* fertilization. In at least one well-known case, a couple divorced after having produced a number of embryos and had them frozen, which led to questions about whose property or responsibility they were. Custody of such embryos, however, though perhaps difficult to establish in a fair way, is hardly on the same plane of social and moral seriousness as custody of children would be. Nor is the decision to dispose of such embryos, whether the parents remain together or not, anything like a decision to dispose of children. It is more like a decision to abort pregnancy in the very early stages, earlier perhaps than therapeutic abortion is normally possible. Singer repeatedly reminds us of our society's commonly accepted beliefs about what is right and wrong in this regard; abortion is generally acceptable to the majority of people, within a wider or narrower range of circumstances and according to the preferences of the parents, which is entirely consistent with allowing parents to do as they please with frozen embryos and on Singer's view even, as we have seen, with very young infants. Reason plays a supporting role, via improved understanding of the beginnings of human life, giving our moral values and precepts a rationale compatible with the facts.

Just as the scientific account of syngamy and twinning has altered our concept of the early stages of a human *being* or individual, so the scientific account of the genetics of our species has altered our concept of what it is to be a *human* being. As we saw earlier, it is now known that our DNA differs from that of chimpanzees by only 1.6%. Put the other way around, humans are 98.4% identical with chimpanzees, genetically. According to Singer, this fact undercuts all "speciesist" claims of decisive human difference from or superiority to chimpanzees or, to a slightly lesser degree, the other great apes. The chimpanzees are our cousins, if not our brothers, and should be treated accordingly. In other words, the respect traditionally accorded to human beings, just because they are human, ought to be extended to chimpanzees and to the other great apes. At issue here is our inclination concerning what we might call "moral proximity." Just as Christians attempt to expand the concept of "neighbor" to include the entire human race, so Singer attempts to expand the circle, as he calls it, of those beings, human and non-human, who are so like us that they should be included when we say "us." A chimpanzee, then, is quite literally "one of us" from a genetic point of view, that is, from the enlightened viewpoint of what I have called experimental reason. The ramifications for ethics are clear; in order to be consistent we must treat the two species of chimpanzees, *Pan troglodytes* and *Pan paniscus*, with the same moral delicacy that we usually reserve to *Homo sapiens*. Again experimental reasoning proves an aid to moral decision-making by ensuring that decisions are made with as full an understanding as possible of the relevant facts.

REPLY TO SINGER ON EXPERIMENTAL REASONING

Indeed the facts about physical reality are important to ethics, and to Singer's credit he is one of those rare philosophers who take such facts seriously, going to the trouble of learning them and applying that factual knowledge in the normative realm. In philosophy, the tradition of respect for the facts extends back to Aristotle (384–322 B.C.E.) and has been upheld by empiricists and utilitarians of whom Singer is one, following in the footsteps of Thomas Hobbes (1588–1679), Jeremy

Bentham, and J.S. Mill. The competing tradition in philosophy extends back to Plato (427–347 B.C.E.) who emphasized what I have called intuitive reason and calculative reason rather than experimental reason. So-called idealists and rationalists have sided with Plato, and among them the most important ethical thinker is Immanuel Kant (1724–1804) who thought that empiricism and utilitarianism actually make ethics impossible. Without entering into this ancient philosophical debate about the importance of experimental reasoning, suffice it to say that the facts and their application often *can* be questioned and sometimes *must* be when the point at issue involves ethics.[4] This is because, as we have noted repeatedly, ethics involves *what ought to be*, not only *what is*, and when we enter the realm of what ought to be we take with us our desires and our will as well as our curiosity and our intellect. In the realm of ethics, even more than in the realm of science (though there, too) we must be careful to avoid simply seeing what we want to see and hearing what we want to hear.

Singer's discussion of the old idea of a "moment of conception" in light of new discoveries concerning syngamy is, I think, a case in point. Because he has set for himself the general goal of showing how traditional morality is inadequate to our times, and how it should be replaced, he sees the scientific evidence in that light, as eliminating the old belief in a moment of conception. But in fact it is just as plausible to view the scientific evidence in another light, namely, as replacing the "moment of conception" with a "moment of syngamy."

For the process factor, so to speak, is the same in both cases. Neither conception nor syngamy is thought of as taking place apart from a series of events, one following after another such that the removal of any one of them will amount to preventing the future existence of one or more human beings. We can think of the series as perhaps bound on one end by some kind of decision in one way or another to allow sperm to be in close enough proximity to an ovum, and at the other end by a decision for or against infanticide. In between, whether we point to conception (penetration of the cell wall of an ovum by a sperm) or to syngamy (joining of genetic material from sperm and ovum) we do indeed have a moment at which *at least one* unique human being begins to exist. Singer even refers to "the moment of syngamy,"[5] acknowledging that at every moment a given instance of syngamy either is or is not complete whether we know of or can actually detect its completeness or not. The simple application of a principle of logic, of what I have called calculative reasoning, shows us that at any given moment a given process either is or is not completed, and there can be no gray area in between in reality *at that moment.*[6] The apparent gray area is only a function of our ignorance. In the same way we can know that a given quantity of salt is at any given moment either completely dissolved or not in a given quantity of water, though we may not be able to tell precisely when it is completely dissolved.

Logic also shows that during the period of time when twinning remains a possibility, when it is as Singer points out not true to say that we have exactly one human being, it does *not* therefore follow that we have no human being. It is entirely possible that what we have in the growing embryo is *at least* one human being, though not yet known to us to be *at most* one human being. In fact, given that we are talking about a human entity post syngamy, with a unique genetic code (in the sense that no other being has it, though perhaps several will if twinning occurs), it seems most reasonable to regard it as a human *being or beings.* Though Singer may admit this last point (and not lose his argument about abortion over it, there being cases when it is permissible to kill an innocent human being in his view), still it is important to him that we not consider the zygote a human individual or individual*s.* I shall have more to say about this in chapters four and five.

For present purposes two points are important. First of all, logic or calculative reasoning serves as a corrective to experimental reasoning in some cases. Where we detect a gray area, for instance, in a physical process, we may wish to sort out the things that admit of gray areas from the things that do not. Being or existence, for example, does not admit of gray areas in the sense that for any given entity and any given moment of time, the entity in question either exists or it does not whether we know of its status as to existence or not.[7] This brings us to the second important point: intuitive reasoning also can check experimental thinking by opening our minds to qualitative and normative dimensions of things lest we become too enchanted with the quantitative and factual. Thus we might well reflect that human zygotes are completely human in a way that skin cells or gametes are not, and by virtue of their humanity we might well say they are not to be trifled with. A certain awe or reverence before the human should temper, for instance, our possible enchantment with the technology of cloning humans.[8]

I think Singer has especially taken leave of his intuitive reasoning on the topic of chimpanzees. No amount of experimental reasoning or quantitative analysis of DNA can ever hope to obviate the very obvious qualitative differences between humans and chimps, or at least, not if we keep our wits about us. It is rather the controlling desire to prove a pervasive similarity between us and them—in Singer's case, for ethical purposes—that can bring us to view ape behavior as virtually human.[9] This despite the undeniable fact that studies of DNA and of primate behavior are *human* activities, not simian ones. The reply to the effect that the apes are watching and perhaps studying us, too, is beside the point; they are closer to turtles than they are to us in terms of the quality of their articulated analysis.

Qualitative distinctions are of huge importance for human thinking generally and for ethics in particular. To the extent that modern science emphasizes the quantitative and neglects the qualitative, then (from a philosophical and ethical perspective) it stands in need of a dose of intuitive reasoning, of appreciation for the categories and values of things.[10]

SINGER ON "RATIONAL INSIGHT" AS AN AID TO ETHICAL THINKING

To be fair, Singer would in one sense not deny this, insofar as his exploration of primate studies is intended to enlighten us about humans' "chimpanzee" nature and about chimpanzees' "human" nature (as he says, we are the "third chimpanzee"). It is in thus "expanding the circle" of our ethical concern that he sees the value to ethics of what I have called intuitive reasoning. There is a fundamental rational insight which, added on to our subjective preferences, renders us ethical beings in the true sense of the term for Singer. What happens is that we begin to see our own preferences as no more important than other people's—first with regard to the people close to us, then with regard to people further removed or even unknown to us, and finally with regard to all sentient creatures. In Singer's words:

When my ability to reason shows me that the suffering of another being is very similar to my own suffering and (in an appropriate case) matters just as much to that other being as my own suffering matters to me, then my reason is showing me something that is undeniably *true*. I can still choose to ignore it, but then I can no longer deny that my perspective is a narrower, and more limited one, than it could be. This may not be enough to yield an objectively true ethical position. (One can always ask: what is so good about having a broader and more all-encompassing perspective?) But it is as close to an objective basis for ethics as there is to find.[11]

Reason thus seems to show us that the like preferences of all sentient creatures ought to be weighed equally, which is a kind of rational insight—rational because universal and objective, and an insight because understood directly rather than being proved by science or by logic. It makes a claim about the categories and values of things, namely that all sentient creatures feel pleasures and pains that matter in some way. But the principle of equal consideration of interests, as this idea is called, is truly a moral or normative principle, and not a mere factual or rational principle. Thus remarkably it is neither true nor false in Singer's view.

This distinction between the moral or normative and the factual or rational is important in this context because, as we have seen, Singer agrees in principle with Hume who taught that "reason is the slave of the passions," in other words, that reason itself does not determine matters of desire and preference in which morality consists. Reason can show that our moral decisions are inconsistent with our moral principles, perhaps, but it cannot in the mere discovery of logical consistency or inconsistency decide what is morally right. How then does Singer arrive at a fundamental moral principle which is inherently rational without violating his own distinction? An illustration may help us to sort this out. Consider the following argument that makes use of preferences (evaluative or normative expressions) in its first premise and in its conclusion, while its second premise is purely a matter of fact:

> Hurray for amphibians!
> Frogs are amphibians.
> Therefore, hurray for frogs![12]

Reason cannot say anything for or against a tendency to praise amphibians as such, just as it cannot on Singer's account say anything for or against any preference. But it can tell us that if we say "Hurray for amphibians and down with frogs," then we are being inconsistent with ourselves. This seems to be something like what Singer is claiming about the position according to which our own preferences matter but those of other sentient beings do not. But the cases are not entirely parallel. We would need to construct two arguments. First an argument in which the first premise and the conclusion contain a fact about preferences, while the second premise is an ordinary "scientific" fact:

> My pleasure and pain matter (to me).
> I am a sentient being.
> Therefore, the pleasures and pains of all sentient beings matter (to them).

Then the second argument would proceed as follows:

> The pleasures and pains of all sentient beings matter to them and ought to be taken into account.
> Chimpanzees (say) are sentient beings.
> Therefore, the pleasures and pains of chimpanzees matter to them and ought to be taken into account.

With this expansion to two arguments I think we can clarify Singer's train of thought with regard to the relation between what I have called intuitive reasoning and ethics. Reason exercises its *calculative function* in the second argument, where it is shown that given the universal premise about sentient creatures' pleasure and pain I am constrained, if I am to be consistent, to acknowledge the value of chimpanzees' pleasure and pain. But reason exercises its *intuitive function* in the first argument where the extension is made from my own pleasure and pain to the pleasure and pain of every sentient creature. This is an insight, rather than strictly a matter of consistency. But it is rational rather than normative because it expresses not a preference, strictly speaking, but a fact about preferences. The normative element is added in to the first premise and conclusion of the second argument to represent the moral point of view that Singer prefers and advocates.

Borrowing an expression from Sidgwick, Singer calls the perspective gained by this rational insight "the point of view of the universe." As he says,

In reasoning about practical matters, we are able to distance ourselves from our own point of view and take on, instead, a wider perspective, ultimately even the point of view of the universe. . . . Reason makes it possible for us to see ourselves this way because, by thinking about my place in the world, I am able to see that I am just one being among others, with interests and desires like others.[13]

Consistent with his view that the foundations of ethics lie in subjective preference, Singer rejects the traditional brand of objective ethics, according to which normative statements may be said to be true about the world. But he adds that, "The possibility of being led, by reasoning, to the point of view of the universe provides as much 'objectivity' as there can be."[14]

REPLY TO SINGER ON RATIONAL INSIGHT

One result of adopting the point of view of the universe is that our obligations to needy people in the third world become as weighty as our obligations to family members who may be in need. After all, Singer's insight is that pain matters, regardless of who feels it, and it would seem to follow that if I can alleviate any pain I ought to do so. Without entering into the debate here about whether our obligations are in fact greater to those who are nearer and dearer to us, it certainly may be admitted that there is a side of Singer's ethics that is very demanding morally and to that extent admirable.

Another result of adopting the point of view of the universe, as we shall see in the next chapter, is that our obligations to non-human animals become far more important than we might otherwise have thought. Again, Singer's insight is that pain matters, regardless of what feels it, and presumably many non-human animals suffer just as human beings do. Thus Singer holds that if we can alleviate the suffering of non-human animals without sacrificing something of comparable value to us, then we should do so.[15] And again, Singer's view is morally demanding and to that extent admirable; perhaps "deep vegetarianism"[16] is a more worthy lifestyle than is the heedless consumption of animal products given the grim realities of factory farming. But with the extension of moral standing to non-human animals we are inevitably led to the question, what is the value of the point of view of the universe? For the question has been answered by Singer in a way that may legitimately be questioned.

Singer has appealed to our regard for universality and objectivity in ethics. But the idea that the moral point of view is universal and objective must specify what it is universal and objective *about* before it can command our assent. For instance, equality before the moral law, though it tends now to be in some vague sense a *prima facie* moral value for most people, is a mere indication of some sort of universality until its extent is specified. Normally, of course, we now take this kind of equality to apply to all *human beings* (though our ancestors may have taken it to apply only to those who owned property). Thus in its regard for universality ordinary modern moral sensibility follows Kant who formulated his famous "categorical imperative" first in a general way and then more specifically. For the first formula of the categorical imperative presented by Kant directs us in general to "Act only according to that maxim by which you can at the same time will that it should become a universal law."[17] This is similar to the lesson parents commonly try to teach their children when they ask, what if everybody did that?[18] But the second formula, Kant's "practical imperative," directs us in particular; "Act so that you treat humanity, whether in your own person or in that of another, always as an end and never as a means only."[19] This is more like the lesson parents commonly try to teach their children when they point out that siblings, friends, and neighbors are people, too. So granted that universality is legitimately, even necessarily, a part of the moral point of view, in the realm of ethics it is a *human* universality that is ordinarily meant.

Not only that, but the humanity that the universal point of view normally bids us value is understood in terms of the subjective experience each of us has of being human. We can imagine parental admonitions corresponding to the categorical and practical imperatives, respectively: "*You* wouldn't like it, if everybody did that," and "Others deserve respect just as *you* do." The objectivity, then, that emerges when we adopt the universal point of view is not objective in the sense of non-subjective. Far from it. The objectivity that emerges when we adopt the universal point of view is, so to speak, objectivity *about* human subjectivity. Indeed, objectivity must always be about *something*—about the results of an experiment, for instance, or about the quality of a musical performance. And the objectivity that is fundamental to ethics is about *the subjective experience of being human*. We assume this is a universal experience, i.e., had by all humans, and we check our moral decisions against this assumption.[20] In this way objectivity—seeing myself as one among others—and universality—granting all human beings the dignity I grant myself—constitute the contribution that what I have called intuitive reasoning makes to ethics. It is not an abstract or contentless contribution, advocating objectivity or universality *as such*, which would have no meaning. Rather it is humanistic because it is reason applied to the realm of ethics which is a realm of human affairs.

All this has little to do with the universe in the sense of the cosmos, of course. So what does Singer mean in quoting Sidgwick to the effect that we ought to adopt the point of view of the *universe?* It is something like what Thomas Nagel has famously called "the view from nowhere."[21] A disinterested, impartial viewpoint is morally enlightened, according to Singer, because it is not tied to the preferences of a single individual. As he says, "Ethics requires us to go beyond our own personal point of view to a standpoint like that of the impartial spectator who takes a universal point of view."[22] But the problem with such a "universal point of view," or "point of view of the universe," is that it has no moral content. This is what Kant noticed when he supplemented the universality of the categorical imperative with the humanism of the practical imperative. Though he claimed the two are logically equivalent, still he thought it necessary to specify that human dignity, the intrinsic value of each human being as an end, is what gives ethics its binding force. We set this aside at our peril. After all, it is only the individual human moral agent who could choose to adopt the universal point of view in the first place. The only way the universal point of view can have any meaning at all is as one human option among many. The cosmos considered in itself is silent and devoid of value.

No doubt Singer realizes this. He certainly is not telling us that the universe is a moral agent having preferences or interests. His claim is more negative: the viewpoint of a single human being is in effect not a moral viewpoint, according to him, nor is that of a class or a race of human beings, nor ultimately is that of the human species. The moral point of view is somehow the universal viewpoint of all sentient beings, all who feel pleasure and pain. But in the end, alas, this is not a viewpoint at all, much less a moral one. Or at best it becomes a viewpoint only when adopted by individual human moral agents, one by one. In sum, all interests and preferences involve an individual point of view, and Singer has told us that ethics involves interests and preferences. Therefore he must admit that ethics inherently involves individual point of view. But if the point of view of the universe *is* a point of view at all, then it is individual, and if it is not individual it is not a moral point of view.

Moreover ethics is not a matter of mere facts, even about what the collective preferences or interests of the universe of sentient beings may be. It is a matter of what each of us human moral agents *should* want. No amount of straw, in the form of preferences that sentient beings *do* have can be spun into the gold of what human moral agents *ought to be*. Yet Singer seems to think that the moral will supervene upon or emerge from the factual, provided the universe of facts is large enough in scope. This seems wildly preposterous, at best.

At worst, it is a dangerous negation of the very thing morality ought to respect and strive to preserve, namely, the individual human point of view. In fact, universality, or universalization, as a test of individual moral choice is designed precisely to uphold the claim of each human individual to dignity and respect. But at Singer's hands it becomes a kind of depersonalization, as though the individual perspective were too narrow to count as a moral one and so the universal perspective must replace it.

This has to be denied. To the contrary, human moral agents are the ones—so far as we know, the only ones—who choose one universe rather than another, and act to make their preferred world a reality repeatedly, deliberately, and often in anguish. The universe may function as an instrument (the test of universalizability) or an object (a preferred world) of human moral decision making and action. But it is not the source or arbiter of moral value.

THE POINT OF VIEW OF THE AGENT

The source and arbiter or moral value, for good or ill, is the individual human moral agent who prefers and chooses one world rather than another, in effect, each time she or he decides what to do. Ultimately this means that the role of reason in ethics is a subordinate one[23] (to this extent I agree with Singer and Hume) because the value of reason is to be found in how well it serves human ends (to this extent I reject Singer's and Hume's emphasis on what *is* preferred in favor of an emphasis on what *ought to be* preferred, thus opening up a distinction between correct and incorrect preference). The several functions of reason delineated above—its calculative, experimental, and intuitive functions, by which it promotes consistency, an understanding of the relevant empirical facts, and a good appreciation of the categories and values of things respectively—are all to be directed toward what promotes our common humanity. In thus subordinating reason to human values I am by implication adopting three controversial positions in contrast to Singer's ethics which constitute the basis of my refutation of his theory.

First, I am saying that when reason does not promote our common humanity then reason must be overruled. Reason is capable, for instance, of lending a specious respectability to all kinds of inhuman schemes, from genocide and "ethnic cleansing" to withholding nourishment and medical care from the poor, the sick, the deformed, the disabled, and the deeply inconvenient. It is not reason but a feeling for her humanity that moves a man to see to it that his elderly mother, who suffers from Alzheimer's, is well cared for. The rational cost-benefit analysis Singer advocates speaks against this, or at best, it notes that nursing home workers are thus kept employed.[24]

On a superficial level, the idea that reason can be overruled in the interests of morality seems to fly in the face of twenty-five hundred years of Western philosophy, according to the traditions of which reason ought always to rule. But at a deeper level, where we notice that this is really *human* reason we are talking about, philosophers from Socrates and Aristotle to David Hume have in one way and another called our attention to the fact that it is individual people and not their arguments that ultimately gain our moral admiration. Thus in Aristotle it is the *spoudaios*, the serious man, who provides the standard of moral virtue and adjudicates questions concerning the real and the apparent good; what *is* good is what *appears* good to him. My suggestion is that we take this one step further and insist that after reason has spoken, after we know what is consistent, scientifically respectable, and in accord with rational understanding, it falls to each of us to decide, for instance, how we shall treat human embryos, fetuses, and infants and how we shall regard the elderly, the infirm, the terminally ill, and the other primates. These decisions and choices are to be made by human individuals, not by rational algorithms, and they are to be made from the point of view of the individual human moral agent, not from the alleged point of view of the universe. Something passes between a man and his mother, rightly so, in which calculative and experimental reason play no role.

Secondly, and as a direct result of the first position, I am saying that there are no ethical principles or theories that we can rely upon to "make moral decisions" for us. This, too, may appear to fly in the face of centuries of tradition in ethics, according to which the important philosophical disputes concern which of several competing ethical theories is the best. In proposing a combination of utilitarianism and Kantianism,[25] R.M. Hare seems to imply that it does not matter which theory is the best, and to a certain extent I agree. But I disagree with both Hare and Singer since I propose that we abandon the project of refining ethical theories and turn instead to questions about what is best for humanity in our day and age. Ancient Greek questions about "the good for man" should be made to live again, while differences between competing theories on whether there are moral absolutes, whether consequences ought to matter, and the like, should be let go. Nobody's life has been made better, while many have been made worse or even ruined, by the tragic human tendency to stick to an alleged moral principle despite obviously pernicious effects, as the blood baths of the twentieth century have amply shown. By the same token, Singer's overemphasis on consequences threatens to cheapen human life.

Thirdly, I take the position that ethics is fundamentally, as Aristotle says, a matter of human friendship. His argument to this effect is worth quoting at some length for it ranges over the whole human realm of ethics, from the bond between parent and child to the relations among fellow citizens:

[T]he affection of parent for child and of child for parent seems to be a natural instinct not only in man but in birds and most animals; and similarly the mutual friendliness between members of the same species, especially of the human species, which is why we commend those who love their fellow men. One can see also in one's travels how near and dear a thing every man is to every other. Friendship also seems to be the bond that holds communities together, and lawgivers seem to attach more importance to it than to justice; because concord seems to be something like friendship, and concord is their primary object—that and eliminating faction, which is enmity. Between friends there is no need for justice, but people who are just still need the quality of friendship; and indeed friendliness is considered to be justice in the fullest sense. It is not only a necessary thing, but a splendid one. We praise those who love their friends, and the possession of many friends is held to be one of the fine things of life. What is more, people think that good men and friends are the same.[26]

Ethics rests on the affection we feel, one on one, for our fellow human beings and on our implicit regard for them and for ourselves. Without this foundation in the flesh all ethical thinking is mere hollow application of principle and mechanical calculation.[27]

These three positions—that reason should sometimes be overruled, that ethical principles and theories are not decisive in moral choice, and that ethics rests on human friendship—follow specifically from the subordination of calculative and experimental reason to a correct intuition of human values. The classic reply however, from the philosophical point of view, is that reason is what makes us moral in the first place, so that to reject it is to be irrational and hence to flirt dangerously with immorality and evil. The idea is that reason and human values are equivalent; the reasonable *is* the good, and the unreasonable or irrational is the bad for human beings. The spirit of Singer's ethical theory is paradoxically consistent with this outlook. Despite all his protests to the contrary in support of Hume's idea that reason is the "slave of the passions," in rejecting the distinctively human point of view in favor of the point of view of the universe Singer is really advocating his own version of the old philosophical idea that the rational is the good, that the rational transcends and ought to transcend the human. Partly he is concerned, as we have seen, that individual human beings take too narrow a sphere into consideration when they make moral decisions. Their own preferences and interests are all that really count; in a word they are selfish, which is the antithesis of being moral. This is why, for Singer, the point of view of the universe leads to the principle of the equal consideration of interests, according to which the like preferences and interests of each sentient being, whether human or non-human, count equally with those of every other. In opposing this by emphasizing the individual point of view, the possible subordination of reason to the human good, and the primacy of human friendship, have I then lapsed into a kind of amoral egoism, in other words, into the view that what I prefer is what is good for me and nobody else really matters unless I want them to? This question, and the role in general of Singer's principle of the equal consideration of interests, will be the subject of chapter four.

NOTES

1. Philosophers will notice that I make no mention of the distinction between theoretical (speculative) reason and practical (moral) reason; but my discussion of reason is not undertaken for its own sake, rather it serves the purpose of shedding light on Singer's ethical theory. Certainly it is possible

to analyze reason in such a way that many more distinctions are made: see G.W.F. Hegel, *Phenomenology of Mind* (various editions), among other sources. And it is also possible to give a simpler account than I do. Maybe what I call experimental reasoning is really just a specific variety of calculative or of intuitive reasoning, and not strictly a third kind of rational activity. My arguments will be unaffected, however, because nothing rests on the kinds of reasoning as such. The point is simply to examine the roles that reason plays in Singer's ethics with a view to asking whether he is right about the results.

2. See *Rethinking Life and Death: The Collapse of Our Traditional Ethics* (New York: St. Martin's Press, 1994), p. 100.

3. See Singer, *Rethinking Life and Death*, pp. 93–100.

4. Part of the reason for this is that experimental reasoning can be guided (or rather, misguided) by preconceived notions of what the conclusion should be: thus the so-called science of craniometry purported to show that members of the white race are more intelligent than members of other races. See Stephen J. Gould's discussions of this and related topics in his *Mismeasure of Man* (New York: Norton, 1981), and *Full House: The Spread of Excellence from Plato to Darwin* (New York: Harmony Press, 1996).

5. *Rethinking Life and Death*, p. 96.

6. The relevant principle is known as "Excluded Middle," according to which, in schematic terms, every thing is either *p* or *not-p*. (This says, not that every thing is either black or white, but that every thing is either black or non-black.) A related principle is known as "Non-contradiction," according to which nothing is both *p* and *not-p*. Though logicians may have an interest in constructing systems of logic which deny the principle of excluded middle, these have perhaps no more application to the world of empirical facts, or to the arena of moral decision making, than non-Euclidean geometries (which deny the parallel postulate) have to engineering projects on the Earth.

7. See R.M. Chisholm, *On Metaphysics* (Minneapolis: University of Minnesota Press, 1989). Part II, chapter 6, "Coming into Being and Passing Away: Can the Metaphysician Help?" The late G.E.M. (Elizabeth) Anscombe is said by her husband, Peter Geach, to have held that, "a theory of ethics without a theory of mind was bound to be bogus." (See Sarah Boxer, "G.E.M. Anscombe, 81, British Philosopher," *The New York Times*, Obituaries, 13 January 2001, p. B15.) It is an underlying presupposition of my critique of Singer's ethical theory that, to paraphrase Anscombe, a theory of ethics without a solid metaphysics is bound to be bogus. The chapter in Chisholm's book on metaphysics was originally published in S.F. Spicker and H.T. Englehardt, Jr., eds., *Philosophical Medical Ethics: Its Nature and Significance* (Dordrecht: D. Reidel Publishing, 1977), as a metaphysical commentary on the fundamental questions about being that underlie debates concerning abortion and the withdrawal of life-support. It is certainly true that in the twentieth century the whole enterprise of metaphysical thinking was called into question and declared by many to be outdated and useless. In

my opinion, however, it remains the indispensable foundation of all philo-sophical inquiry, not in the sense that any particular metaphysical theory will ever be accepted by all as the one true theory, but rather in the sense that thinking carefully about metaphysical issues is essential to clear philosophical thinking in other areas, including ethics. My insistence in chapters four and five that Singer is in error when he categorizes sentient beings according to their cognitive attributes rather than according to their species (the kinds of beings they in fact are) stems from metaphysical reflection on the distinction between a being and its attributes.

8. In this way, then, there may be a kind of system of "checks and bal-ances" among the several functions of reason, so that none charges off with-out leave from the others; for admittedly experimental reasoning also provides a reality check when calculative reasoning imposes the requirements of logic illegitimately on physical reality, and when intuitive reasoning mis-takes what *ought to be* for what *is* the case. The first kind of error would occur, for instance, if calculative reasoning were to insist that all swans are white just because all the swans we've experienced so far are white, so that when some black ones turn up in New Zealand they are automatically thought not to be swans. The second kind of error would occur if intuitive reasoning were to conclude that all humans should have the same cholesterol levels or blood pressure in order to be healthy, whereas in fact there is a fairly wide range of normal.

9. Others are motivated by research interests, for instance, to prove that because they are like us non-human primates can be taught to make change. Singer argues in the reverse direction, because they can make change, there-fore they are like us and should be treated with the same respect as humans.

10. Again, I do not specifically distinguish here between theoretical (or speculative) uses of reason and practical (or moral) uses.

11. *How Are We to Live? Ethics in an Age of Self-Interest* (Amherst, NY: Prometheus Books, 1995), pp. 231–232.

12. I owe this delightful and very useful example to my colleague, Prof. Joseph Spoerl.

13. *How Are We to Live?*, p. 229.

14. Ibid., p. 231.

15. See Singer, *Animal Liberation*, chapter six, "Speciesism Today," pp. 213–248, and "The Singer Solution to World Poverty," *The New York Times Magazine*, 5 September 1999, pp. 60–63.

16. See Ian Hacking, "Our Fellow Animals," (review of J.M. Coetzee, *The Lives of Animals* and Peter Singer, *Ethics Into Action: Henry Spira and the Animal Rights Movement*) in *The New York Review of Books*, 29 June 2000, pp. 20–26. "Deep vegetarianism" is more than a lifestyle option ac-cording to which a vegan diet is required along with denial of human unique-ness. It involves concern for animals as such, and becomes a moral and philo-sophical way of life. As Hacking points out, wearing leather shoes or belts is

sharply inconsistent with deep vegetarianism—an expression he borrows from Michael Fox's book, *Deep Vegetarianism* (Temple University Press, 1999).

17. Immanuel Kant, *Foundations of the Metaphysics of Morals*, trans. Lewis White Beck (Indianapolis: Bobbs-Merrill,1959, 1976), p. 39. Singer is a utilitarian, of course, and not a Kantian at all. But on the issue of universality in ethics Kant is the most eloquent source, and in any event, universal principles including Singer's require specification of content, whether they are empiricist or rationalist, deontological or utilitarian in their character as part of a system.

18. Kant's formula is similar but not identical to the parental question because Kant is interested, not in possible obnoxious consequences of a bad maxim, but rather in its inherent inconsistency.

19. Ibid., p. 47.

20. For the moment I set aside questions about infants, the mentally impaired, the comatose, and so on, but will take them up again in chapters four and five.

21. See his book of that title (Oxford University Press, 1986).

22. Singer, *Practical Ethics*, p. 317.

23. By "reason" in this context and throughout the rest of the book I mean, primarily, what I have called "calculative reason" and "experimental reason." But what I have called "intuitive reason" is also to be included to the extent that it lacks content, as I think it does in Singer's treatment. For this reason I say inclusively that reason should be subordinated to human concerns, and I thereby sacrifice philosophical precision for purposes of rhetorical clarity. The effect I anticipate is that philosophers will rightly object that intuitive reason properly understood (whether in the theoretical realm or in the practical realm) *includes* a correct apprehension of the human good. On the other hand, lay readers will likely understand that when I say reason should be subordinated to human values I mean that the rationality of logic and science is not enough to guarantee that human values will be respected. The deeper question about the relation between reason and emotion, or intellect and will, in the area of ethics remains. I think that the work done in neurology by Antonio Damasio and others, though it may not completely resolve the question, nevertheless does shed important light to this extent: it shows fairly conclusively that emotion and reason are more intertwined and interdependent than previous scientific and philosophical analyses have quite appreciated. Ordinary common sense and traditional philosophy may in fact be open to these empirical findings to the extent that they already distinguish between information and knowledge, and between knowledge and wisdom. If the emotional component is not obvious to us in the processing of information or in the acquisition of knowledge (though Damasio finds it there, too), it certainly is obvious to us in the wisdom of those who actually know how to live a good life.

24. See Michael Specter, "The Dangerous Philosopher," *The New Yorker*, September 6, 1999, pp. 46–55.

25. See Hare, "Why I am Only a Demi-Vegetarian," in Dale Jamieson, ed., *Singer and his Critics* (Oxford: Blackwell, 1999), pp. 233–246.

26. Aristotle, *Ethics*, Book VIII, 1155a-b, trans. J.A.K. Thomson, rev. Hugh Tredennick, intro. Jonathan Barnes (London: Penguin, 1976), pp. 258–259.

27. For an eloquent, "continentalist" treatment of this topic, see John Caputo, *Against Ethics* (Bloomington and Indianapolis: Indiana University Press, 1993), especially chapter nine, "Jewgreek bodies: An Antiphenomenological Supplement to the Lyrical-Philosophical Discourses," pp. 194–219. This is an extended meditation on *hyle* (matter), *morphe* (form), body, flesh, touching and being touched, as these relate to our sense of ethical community.

Chapter Four

The Principle of Equal Consideration of Interests

As we noted in chapter one, Singer sees it as a primary goal of philo-sophical ethics to establish a fundamental ethical principle. Before turn-ing to a discussion of the meaning and ramifications of Singer's proposed fundamental ethical principle, let us briefly review what we have said so far about his ethical theory.

To begin with, we saw that Singer believes we should not put much stock in our basic moral intuitions because they are tainted at the source. That is to say, much of what we find to be customary, accept-able, and right behavior is in fact nothing more than the result of natu-ral selection. Kin preference, and even the genuine concern for others as distinct from mere pretense, have had survival value throughout the history of our species, but no normative or ethical claim follows from these facts. Reason shows us that a moral principle is something quite different from a biological adaptation.

Beyond basic moral intuitions which all humans may share due to their presumptive biological basis, Singer also finds fault with our tradi-tional morality in the West. Our acceptance of the principle of the sanc-tity of human life, for instance, is "one of the relics of our cultural history to place alongside the relics of our evolutionary history."[1] Traditionally, this principle has been employed to answer questions about the morality of taking human life under all kinds of circumstances, but according to Singer we can see its uselessness now in an age of organ transplants and advanced medical knowledge about irreversible loss of various brain functions. Moreover, the principle of the sanctity of *human* life is tantamount to speciesism, a morally reprehensible stance comparable to racism or sexism. Given our knowledge of the capacities and behaviors of many non-human animals it is time to relinquish the moral tradition based upon belief in human uniqueness.

Thus, for Singer, there is no hope of finding the fundamental ethical principle in either our moral intuitions or our traditional morality, for neither biological adaptation nor cultural norms can provide a genuine, rationally defensible foundation for ethics. But as we also noted, it is not clear that Singer has established *his* claims about moral intuition and about traditional morality. For the logical independence of fact and value is such that even if it is true that kin preference, for example, is a biological adaptation, from this fact alone it would not follow that kin preference is not the basis of a legitimate moral principle (namely, that our moral obligations are greater to those who are near and dear than to those more remote from us). It may well be such a legitimate basis, or it may not be, but biological adaptation says nothing about the answer to that question. Likewise, the fact that some moral principle, say the sanctity of human life, is part of traditional morality in the West, or that it is hard to apply today, does not debunk it as a legitimate moral principle. It may well be such a legitimate principle, or it may not be, but its factual status as a traditional belief, or as currently hard to apply, says nothing about the answer to that question.

In fact, as we noted, it may well be that some moral intuitions (such as kin preference) and some principles of traditional morality (such as the sanctity of human life) are actually indispensable to a genuinely humane moral code. If this is true, since it is a moral claim, it is true regardless of the facts about the sources of the relevant intuitions or principles.

Next we saw that Singer pursues the separation between facts and values all the way to the root of the concept of moral value. For him, the fact/value distinction somewhat parallels the objective/subjective distinction, such that the attribution of moral value becomes an irreducibly subjective phenomenon. "Ethics is no part of the universe, in the way that atoms are,"[2] he tells us, and ultimately, in agreement with David Hume, "reason is the slave of the passions." To Singer, this means that the only legitimate source of moral value is subjective preference. Thus he proposes "preference utilitarianism" as the most reasonable ethical theory: subjective preference itself is beyond the purview of reason, but in the end reason leads us to base ethics on a proper consideration and weighing of subjective preferences. "According to preference utilitarianism, an action contrary to the preference of any being is, unless this preference is outweighed by contrary preferences, wrong."[3] In Singer's version of the theory, special status is granted to "persons," those beings who are "highly future-oriented in their preferences," but the preferences of all sentient beings count—the view we shall discuss in detail shortly.

In Singer's view, as we saw, his preference utilitarianism is a very practical and applicable ethical theory, an advantageous alternative to theories that rely on supposedly objective principles which people cannot agree about and which are unsuited to modern times. But we also saw that there is good reason to regard subjective preference as susceptible to objective evaluation; everyone knows that all subjective preferences are not equally good, and the introduction of criteria of correct and incorrect preference seems morally required at some level. Singer is therefore wrong to exclude all objectivity from the foundation of ethics. Moreover, some subjective preferences may be inherently correct and indispensable to all other genuinely moral principles and judgments, for instance, the preference that grants intrinsic value to human life. Finally, we saw that the moral life is lived precisely in that area of anxiety and even anguish over how to apply a principle such as the sanctity of human life in specific cases. Singer's attempt to defuse the anguish, though understandable (who really likes anguish?) is wrong-headed. Not that needless anguish brought about by ignorance of the facts or by an overly scrupulous conscience has any value in itself, but rather, the countenanced violation of a high moral principle ought to cause anguish no matter what the agent's ultimate decision—as when a soldier hesitates before killing his fatally wounded comrade whose last cries of agony rend the heart.

Ethical choice plays out in the battlefield of life, and it is serious business. Singer rightly recommends that we go forth armed with a knowledge of the relevant facts and with that expansive and charitable vision which sees in others' interests something as important to them as our interests are to us. But as we saw, what Singer makes of the scientific facts and of the "point of view of the universe" is a coldly value-neutral world in which scientific facts displace moral values and the legitimate point of view of the individual human being is delegitimated and even morally erased. Properly speaking, neither of these developments should have occurred in his system, given the logical separation of facts and values with which Singer began. Be that as it may, let me repeat that no scientific fact—about the beginning of life, or about the boundaries of our species, for instance—can acquire an appropriate moral application apart from the moral viewpoint that belongs specifically and rightfully to individual human beings, in the flesh, who do and ought to value and prize above all else other individual human beings.

Given this critique of Singer's views so far, I noted that my view in opposition to Singer rests on three basic claims: (1) in ethics reason must be subordinated to the human good, as understood in the classic sense of that which concerns and motivates the morally admirable among us; (2) there are no ethical theories or principles or algorithms or calculi that can "make our moral decisions for us"—each of us is "the man on the ground," at the interface between principle and specific situation, whenever we make a moral choice; and (3) ethics is fundamentally a matter of human affection and friendship, in the sense that without this there would neither be, nor be a need for, ethical thinking. Only this amicable feeling makes us care about our obligations to one another, which is ultimately what stands between us and the absolute domination of warfare and economics.

SINGER'S PRINCIPLE OF EQUAL CONSIDERATION AND ITS RAMIFICATIONS

In concluding chapter three, I suggested that for all his apparent subordination of reason to subjective preference, Singer's emphasis on calculative and experimental reason combined with the emptiness of his intuitive reason makes him in fact an extreme rationalist within the broader tradition of Western thought. Typically, the champions of reason have held that it alone can prevent rampant selfishness and the triumph of barbarism by widening the sphere of our moral concerns. I had indicated that we would check whether Singer's program in fact does what his proposal of the principle of equal consideration of interests promises. Does it provide an improvement over classical conceptions of the human good, ordinary moral intuition, and traditional morality, as he claims?

Singer's rationale for the principle of equal consideration of interests is relatively simple. He has articulated it clearly in *Animal Liberation* and in *Practical Ethics*. Let us take a look at what he says.

Animal Liberation is the earlier work, first published in 1975, with a revised edition appearing in 1990.[4] Chapter one is entitled, "All Animals Are Equal . . . or why the ethical principle on which human equality rests requires us to extend equal consideration to animals too." Very early on he makes the remarkable claim that, "We would be on shaky ground if we were to demand equality for blacks, women, and other groups of oppressed humans while denying equal consideration to non-humans."[5] The reason for this is that the moral principle of human equality is not based on actual equality of human beings; it is not a factual claim to the effect that human beings *are* equal, rather it is a moral prescription to the effect that human beings *ought to receive* equal consideration. As he says it, "Equality is a moral idea, not an assertion of fact." In tracing the moral tradition behind the principle of equality, showing its pedigree, he cites Jeremy Bentham ("Each to count for one and none for more than one") and Henry Sidgwick ("The good of any one individual is of no more importance, from the point of view [if I may say so] of the Universe, than the good of any other"). Thus it is because all humans ought to receive equal consideration that it is wrong to single out male or female, black or white, intelligent or unintelligent for special treatment. The universalizing function of intuitive reason leads us to understand this, as we saw in chapter three. And because the principle of equal consideration of interests is understood in utilitarian terms as the demand that interests, preferences, pleasures, and pains of all should count equally, it quickly follows that "all" in this context must mean "all sentient creatures." For it is all and only sentient creatures who are able to feel pleasure and pain and are thus able to have preferences and interests.

It has been a fundamental concern of Singer's ethical theory from the beginning that the interests of non-human animals be included in human ethical deliberations. Because I think ethics is exclusively a human domain, and legitimately so, I have not dwelt much on Singer's contributions to the Animal Liberation movement. But it must be admitted that it is impossible to understand what he means by the principle of equal consideration of interests apart from this connection. Whenever he applies the principle in the realm of human affairs, or explores its human ramifications, the extension of moral consideration to non-human animals is an indispensable presupposition.

Thus in the later work, *Practical Ethics*, which was first published in 1978 and went into a second edition in 1993,[6] chapter two, "Equality and Its Implications," immediately precedes the chapter entitled, "Equality for Animals?" in which the principle of equality gets its most fundamental explanation in terms of the moral equality of all sentient beings. As in *Animal Liberation*, Singer is again at pains to point out that the moral equality of humans is not based on a factual equality which clearly does not exist. Human beings are obviously unequal in the factual sense, in intelligence and all kinds of other endowments including consciousness, rationality, free agency, and other attributes that may be associated with moral standing in one way or another. Not only that, but some non-human animals are better endowed in these and other ways than some humans are, which forces us to see that sentience "is the only defensible boundary of concern for the interests of others."[7] Because he doubts, "that there is any morally significant property that all humans possess equally,"[8] Singer concludes that the morally significant property shared by all sentient beings, granting it exists in varying degrees, namely their capacity to feel pleasure and pain, is what provides a proper scope for the universalizing impulse of moral reasoning. Thus he declares the principle of equal consideration of interests to be the ultimate basis of all legitimate ethical judgments, the essence of it being, "that we give equal weight in our moral deliberations to the like interests of all those affected by our actions."[9] Application of the principle, according to Singer, will lead not in a simplistic way to equality of treatment, but rather to fairness all things considered:

> The principle of equal consideration of interests acts like a pair of scales, weighing interests impartially. True scales . . . take no account of *whose* interests they are weighing.[10]

In effect, Singer's goal has been to set up this pair of scales, his contribution to ethical theory, one purpose of which in his view is to establish a fundamental ethical principle. By using his scales he hopes to overthrow traditional Western morality and institute his "Copernican Revolution" in ethics. The best way to understand the principle of equal consideration of interests is to examine its ramifications as they play out in the "new commandments" that Singer proposes to replace what he takes to be the old ones.

Singer sums up the essentials of traditional Western morality in five basic "commandments" and in response to them he proposes five new, revised commandments. Let us take a look at each of these in turn, as explained by Singer in his *Rethinking Life and Death: The Collapse of Our Traditional Ethics*, which appeared in 1994.[11]

The first old commandment is, "Treat all human life as of equal worth." Presumably this underlies the traditional "sanctity of human life ethic." The idea is that every human life has intrinsic value and dignity, regardless of any circumstances. In Singer's view, however, almost nobody seriously believes this. Moreover, advances in modern medicine have forced us to admit that in fact all human life is not of equal worth. An anencephalic infant, for instance, or an adult in a persistent vegetative state, do not live lives worth the same as the lives of normal infants or adults. The fact that with modern medical knowledge we can keep them alive does not confer value on the lives of the severely incapacitated. Rather it should prompt us to rewrite the command as follows: "Recognize that the worth of human life varies." This is Singer's first new commandment. It is intended to inform application of the scales provided by the principle of equal consideration of interests. Human life, that is to say, may be weighed in the scales, and its claims may upon occasion be outweighed by competing concerns, rather than the value of human life being treated as a kind of absolute against which other considerations are weighed, itself outweighed by nothing. In Singer's view, weighing human life in the scales frees us up to make beneficial decisions about severely disabled infants and adults, as well as about those who are wholly or partially brain dead. Questions about competing claims for resources can be asked, and answered fairly in a manner that respects the interests of all involved, once we cease maintaining the fiction that a human life of whatever quality has a value equal to that of any other human life.

The principle of equal consideration of interests thus forms the foundation for a coherent ethic applicable to modern biomedical circumstances. Strictly speaking, anencephalic infants, persons in persistent vegetative states, and the brain dead have no interests, inasmuch as they are incapable of feeling pleasure or pain. Questions of life or death for them, then, must be answered in terms of the interests of those who are capable of feeling pleasure and pain and thus of having interests. Once we admit it is not true that all human lives are of equal worth, we can place human life in the balance, so to speak, and analyze the costs and probable outcomes, the burdens and benefits, of the various courses of action that purport to prolong, to enhance, to diminish, or even to end human life.

The second old commandment according to Singer is, "Never intentionally take innocent human life." The intentional taking of innocent human life has traditionally been thought wrong—add malice aforethought and you have a standard definition of murder. But we have seen that for Singer not all human lives are of equal value, and that some are even of such low quality as not to be worth the effort of sustaining them, neither to the individuals themselves nor to their family, friends, or society. Thus we are led to admit that the traditional prohibition against taking innocent human life has no place in a coherent, modern ethical system. Singer therefore proposes a second new commandment in its place: "Take responsibility for the consequences of your decisions." At first blush this may appear to be no more than what any minimal morality, traditional or modern, would recommend. But the context is crucial. Given the advent of modern medical technology and its devices for life-support, the distinction between "killing" and "letting die" has assumed new importance as traditional morality tries to keep pace. The moral distinction between acts and omissions is a long-standing one, but once the decision had to be faced whether to "pull the plug" on life-support, or not, the clash between the old sanctity of human life ethic and modern medicine made this difference crucial. According to Singer, without it the sanctity of human life ethic collapses. For as he points out, whether you decide to withdraw life-support or to administer a lethal injection, the intended outcome for the patient is the same. Honesty about this, he holds, is preferable to the subterfuge, as he sees it, of "letting nature take its course" (just as honesty about live organ donors is preferable, in his view, to the subterfuge, as he sees it, of "brain death"). Hence his second commandment, "Take *responsibility* for the consequences of your *decisions*" (my emphasis). Deciding not to feed or hydrate or provide antibiotics or surgery or intubation and a respirator to a patient, that is, deciding to let the patient die, has the same result as deciding to give the patient a lethal injection. (The lethal injection may in fact be more merciful.) If, as often happens, parents and medical staff agree not to treat or nourish an infant with *spina bifida* or Down's syndrome, that is tantamount to deciding to kill it, since the easily foreseen outcome will be the infant's death. According to Singer, there can be a variety of good reasons to make such a decision, as well as perhaps good reasons to accomplish the objective instead by means of a lethal drug dose, since that could minimize pain. In any event, he would have us renounce the fiction that when we *do something* or take action we are more responsible for the outcome than when we *do nothing* or omit some action. For we are responsible for the outcome either way. The old commandment invites evasions, the new one purports to be more honest.

The third old commandment according to Singer is "Never commit suicide and never assist anyone else in doing so." The spirit of the old commandment is an absolute preference for life, regardless of the circumstances, such that even in cases of terminal illness and severe pain, the value of human life should be sustained and choosing death before natural death would have occurred is not a legitimate option. Singer proposes replacing this with his third new commandment, "Respect a person's desire to live or die." Crucial to this commandment is the underlying distinction between persons and non-persons. Recall that for Singer this distinction is not equivalent to that between humans and non-humans, rather there are actually four categories in the complete account: human persons, non-human persons (such as the great apes), human non-persons (such as infants and severely incapacitated adults), and non-human non-persons (including animals without self-awareness and future-orientation). Both human and non-human persons should be allowed freely to decide whether they wish to live or die, because persons are uniquely those who have a right to life. For non-persons, life and death decisions may be made according to the preferences of others, since they have no preferences themselves, apart from the preference to avoid pain. Thus we should sustain or end the lives of non-persons in such a way that they do not suffer, but whether they are human or non-human should be of no concern to us. For persons, however, who are self-aware and oriented to the future, life and death decisions should be made according to their preferences, and equally so whether they wish to live or to die. Thus assisted suicide, as recently decriminalized in the Netherlands, is in keeping with Singer's third new commandment, as are so-called "active" and "passive" euthanasia, whenever respectful of a person's freely expressed desire. Likewise, assuming the ones whose lives are ended are non-persons, infanticide and euthanizing of the severely incapacitated are in keeping with this commandment so long as the preferences of any persons affected are properly weighed and care is taken not to inflict pain on any sentient creature. Thus an infant who is not yet a person, or an elderly patient who had been a person but now is no longer self-aware and future-oriented, may be killed without violating Singer's commandments. In short, we must respect the desire of any human or non-human person who wishes to live, and those who wish to die may be assisted in this.

The fourth old commandment selected by Singer for replacement is, "Go forth and multiply." This biblical injunction may have had its place, he concedes, in former times when human populations were much smaller. But with today's overpopulation we see that the old commandment has outlived its usefulness. In its stead Singer proposes his fourth new commandment, "Bring children into the world only if they are wanted." The interests to be considered when it comes to the question whether to bring more people into the world are of course those of the people who are already here. Clearly zygotes, embryos, fetuses, and even young infants have no interests to be consulted except the minimal interest in a pain-free existence. Singer points out that this means strictly-speaking that they cannot be harmed, for they have no future-oriented preferences the satisfaction of which could be taken away. Thus what emerges from the fourth new commandment in conjunction with the others and against the backdrop of the equal consideration of interests is a coherent picture including the permissibility of abortion at all stages of pregnancy, and infanticide (by act or omission) at least in early infancy, to the end that every child who is allowed to live is a child that is wanted by its parents or by other interested adults. If the life of a fetus or infant is precious that is purely because its parents or other interested adults see it that way. The value, that is to say, of new human life is not something inherent in it, but rather something attributed to it by persons whose interests are to be weighed with the like interests of others. So, for instance, if a child is very much wanted by its parents, then its life should be protected accordingly. But if the parents do not want it, and if prospects for adoption are not a factor, then the fetus or infant may be disposed of accordingly in some painless way. Again, if the parents really want a child whose condition requires very costly or uncertain medical treatment, then that cost or uncertainty must be weighed in the balance along with parents' interests and those of the larger society. On the other hand, if parents do not want a child even whose medical treatment is relatively inexpensive and reliable, and if adoption is not a factor, then it is morally permissible to withhold treatment and even actively to bring about death according to Singer's new commandments.

The fifth and final old commandment that Singer seeks to replace is, "Always place the highest value on human life because it is human." As we have seen in some detail already, Singer does not grant special value to human life as such. According to the principle of equal consideration of interests, sentient creatures are all fundamentally equal because of their shared capacity to feel pleasure and pain. Moreover, scientific advances in genetics have shown us that human beings are not unique, as had been believed, but rather that the differences among species are differences of degree and not of kind. A normal adult chimpanzee has far more of the features formerly attributed exclusively to human beings, such as self-awareness and communication and computation skills, than a human infant or a retarded human adult. So the basis for giving priority to human concerns because they are human has vanished, according to Singer. Moreover we now see in light of this that "speciesism" is just as morally reprehensible as racism or sexism. Therefore it is Singer's new commandment, "Do not discriminate on the basis of species," that carries moral weight, given our new understanding. Singer quotes the poet, Henry Wadsworth Longfellow, to the effect that "every human heart is human," and refutes the claim. Not every human heart is human, he explains, because the term 'human' has been used equivocally. In its first instance, "every *human* heart is human," it means "member of the species *Homo sapiens*," but in its second instance, "every human heart is *human*," it means "self-aware, compassionate, sensitive," all traits that *do* belong to some non-members of the species *Homo sapiens* and that *do not* belong to some members of the species *Homo sapiens*. We are commanded, therefore, not to discriminate on the basis of species.

Singer readily admits that his new commandments may need to be revised, too. Nevertheless he sees them as a step in the right direction and recommends their application to tough cases that have only proved disabling to the traditional morality of the old commandments. Let us briefly list Singer's principles, and then show how they serve to solve moral dilemmas, how they collectively expose the fundamental weakness of traditional morality, and how they constitute as he claims a Copernican revolution in ethics. After that we shall see how Singer's proposal may be criticized.

Singer's new ethics is essentially constituted by one fundamental moral principle and five moral rules or commandments, as follows:

Principle: The like interests of all sentient creatures that would be affected are to be weighed equally when making moral decisions.

Rule 1: Recognize that the value of human life varies.

Rule 2: Take responsibility for the consequences of your decisions.

Rule 3: Respect a person's desire to live or die.

Rule 4: Bring children into the world only if they are wanted.

Rule 5: Do not discriminate on the basis of species.

Consider first the case of an anencephalic infant whose organs might save the life of an infant with a normal brain. Singer says that according to traditional morality, which values all human life equally and prohibits actions directed at taking innocent human life, it would be wrong to remove a vital organ from an anencephalic infant in order to save the life of the infant with a normal brain. Even the distinction between acts and omissions cannot obscure the fact that to remove an infant's heart is to kill it, regardless of any other good consequences to any other individuals. But Singer's new ethics, especially with rules 1 and 2, makes it plain that one may with a clear conscience judge that the anencephalic baby's life is of relatively little worth, and that killing it is not only generally permissible but morally required in the case where another life can thereby be saved.

Next consider a woman in a persistent vegetative state brought about by some trauma who turns out to be pregnant. Singer says that according to traditional morality it would be morally required to keep the woman's body alive as long as possible in order to give her fetus a chance at life. He also says, though, that most people recoil at this ghoulish prospect in the absence of some overriding preference on the part of the baby's father or the mother's family. Considered as their child or grandchild, the unborn fetus may have some value, but not apart from that in common opinion, as Signer sees it. So his new commandments free us up from the unreasonable requirements of the old commandments, and accord better with what most of us believe. Considering especially rules 1 and 4, we can see that there is no need to sustain the lives of the comatose mother and the unborn child whose mother is incapable of wanting it. The father or the mother's family may decide on the basis of their own preferences either to sustain the pregnancy or to end the lives of both mother and baby without violating Singer's fundamental principle or basic moral rules.

Suppose again that an infant has been born into a situation where there are no adults willing to care for it, either because the infant is so disabled, or else because the adults have died or been severely injured or for other reasons completely lack the resources required of parents. Traditional morality would require that such an infant be fostered and even treasured in some way regardless of impossible circumstances. But Singer's rules 1, 2, 4, and 5 cast a fresh light. The infant's life has no inherent value, but rather is worth just what the concerned adults take it to be. The infant itself cannot be harmed because it has no more conscious prospects for the future than a snail. The fact that it is a human non-person does not mean we should treat it any differently than we would a non-human non-person. But no one sees a moral problem with euthanizing kittens or puppies, say, for which there are no good homes (until their numbers become too great, the majority regard this as sensible and compassionate). From Singer's point of view if we are reasonable we will treat human infants the same. Except for public sentiment which may not be ready for this, he sees no barrier to the moral permissibility of infanticide during some appropriate period of time, perhaps the first month or so after birth.[12]

At the other end of the life span, consider the case of an elderly cancer patient who foresees and dreads the final weeks or months of severe and unremitting pain or unacceptable loss of physical independence. The traditional view has been that it is always wrong to hasten death except in a very limited way as the anticipated but unintended side-effect of certain kinds of pain management. Singer's new commandments however are considerably more lenient and, he would add, humane. In view of rules 1, 2, 3, and 5 we can see that quality of life considerations may be decisive without any violation of proper moral values. First of all, as we have seen, there is no morally significant difference between killing (by lethal injection, say) and letting die (by withholding treatment). Pain killers may legitimately be administered with the intent to hasten death as well as with the intent to relieve pain. Secondly, as the value of human life varies, so does the subjective assessment of that value, hence the need to respect a person's desire to die. Finally, our society is kinder to non-human than to human animals when it comes to old age and infirmity, for we require suffering and forbearance of elderly and infirm humans that we would never impose on a dog. In essence, we are guilty of reverse discrimination on the basis of species. But Singer's new morality would replace the duty to live on in pain with the right to die when one wishes to do so.

According to Singer, the old ethic deals badly with these kinds of difficult cases largely because it has made two fundamental mistakes. The first of these is the spurious distinction between acts and omissions, the second is the priority granted to members of the species *Homo sapiens*. All the dysfunctions of the old morality are traceable to one or the other of these two errors and the success of his proposed new morality will be traceable to their correction. For in every case where we agonize—the doctor could save a baby if he were not forbidden to kill another, badly disabled baby—or where we feel that what morality requires just cannot be rationally justified, we find in the background the old, nearly superstitious ideas that acting is vastly different from refraining to act, or that humans in whatever condition are vastly different from members of any other species of animal. Take these old beliefs away and things clear up. What it is permissible to allow it is also permissible to bring about. Humans may be treated as well as other animals, and *vice versa*.

The world as it would look minus the underlying errors of the old morality and its commandments is what Singer envisions as the beneficial result of his Copernican revolution in ethics. The errors will be increasingly unacceptable to thinking, modern people, and as vestiges of an outworn religious ideology they will simply slip away. At the same time, the pressures from modern medical science and technology will so alter the human world that it would be impossible to sustain the old mo-

rality even if its errors could somehow be swept under the rug. The redefinition of death by the Harvard Committee in 1967 shows the
mechanism here; where the old morality's "sanctity of human life"
clashes with the new technology's facility of organ transplantation,
something has to give. And the British judges who ruled for a "quality of
life" ethic in the case of Tony Bland[13] have shown the spirit and direction
of movement of the new moral outlook. Some human lives are not worth
living. And some of the things we once refused to do even to enhance a
human life will now become commonly accepted. As Singer says, it is not
a question *whether* the old morality will be replaced, but *when* and by
what. His proposals, based on the principle of equal consideration of interests, are not above reproach, however, as we shall shortly see.

REPLY TO SINGER ON THE ETHIC OF EQUAL
CONSIDERATION OF INTERESTS

The principle of equal consideration of interests is Singer's formula
intended to satisfy the requirement of reason that moral norms be universally applicable. But universality itself is a bare logical consideration,
as we noted in chapter three, until it is given some content. As we saw,
Immanuel Kant (1724–1804) gave his universal basic principle (the
categorical imperative) *human* content (the practical imperative). By
contrast, Singer supplies content with the category of *all sentient creatures*. In other words, his principle of equal consideration is in more
precise terms the principle of the equal consideration of the like interests of all sentient creatures. One effect of this, as a departure from traditional morality, is essentially to replace the intrinsic value of a
distinctive *being*, a human being, with the instrumental value of some
of its *attributes*, for instance the ability to feel pleasure and pain. Sentient creatures are obviously benefited by their ability to feel pleasure
and pain; it enhances their prospects for survival by prompting them to
pursue what is advantageous to them and to avoid what is disadvanta-
geous to them. But the ability to feel pleasure and pain is an attribute
not itself valuable apart from the being of the creature that has the ability. Its ability to feel pleasure and pain, for example, is valuable to a
horse for preserving and enjoying its equine existence. The value, then,
is to be found primarily in being a horse, and only subordinately to that
in feeling pleasure or pain as such. Likewise a human's ability to feel
pleasure and pain is valuable to a human for the preservation and enjoy-
ment of human existence. Again, the value is to be found primarily in
being a human, not just in feeling pleasure or pain as such. In fact there

is no sensing of pleasure or pain that is not the attribute or activity of a specific animal of a given kind. Thus Singer's attempt to give content to his fundamental ethical principle by saying that it applies to all sentient creatures as such is unsuccessful. We are still left wondering *whose* pleasure and pain are to be valued as morally significant and why.

Of course, Singer believes there is no morally relevant characteristic that all humans share except for the ability to feel pleasure and pain, which is why he "expands the circle" of ethical concern to include all sentient creatures. In this, however, I think he misapprehends the fundamental nature of ethics, namely, that it is necessarily a *human* concern, and that its guiding impulse is the extension of moral consideration to each and every member *of our own species.* This means, among other things, that morality is a matter not of morally relevant *characteristics* but of morally relevant *entities.* Insofar then as we extend moral consideration to non-human animals, resolving to treat them "humanely," we do so in recognition more of our humanity than of their sentience. We see ourselves, in other words, as creatures who care how we treat those outside our species, a distinctively if not universally human trait.

So unlike Singer, I would like to locate the primary source of moral value in a specific kind of entity, the human being. As we have seen in chapter two, however, Singer holds that the only source of moral value is subjective preference, the subjective preferences of all sentient creatures being basically of equal value. This strikes me as highly implausible. Subjective preference is in reality a human concept; certainly for the human audience Singer addresses it is laden with the connotations he intends of non-objectivity, non-absoluteness, of relative value. That is to say, subjective preference is understood to be the personal preference of one rational, self-aware human being among others. Is the hawk's "preference" for a mouse like this? If we credit non-human animals with having such preferences it is because they approximate the human in specifiable ways, not because, as Singer would have it, we cannot clearly distinguish between them and us.

Singer's principle of the equal consideration of interests, read as equal consideration of the like interests of all sentient creatures, seems to me illicitly to override the fundamentally human nature of subjective preference. In other words, it bids us consider the preferences of all sentient creatures, whether human or not, as if they were human preferences, and then declares the precedence traditionally granted the human to be morally illegitimate. In the end, rather than raising our level of concern for non-human animals, it lowers our regard for everything human. I noted earlier in this chapter that Singer's principle of equal consideration is best understood through his expansion of it into the five "new commandments." My critique of his principle will likewise be clearer in this light. My general contention is that, given our changing world of advances in technology and medicine, what we need is to re-establish human values, not to overthrow them as Singer proposes.

Singer's first new commandment, that we recognize that the worth of human life varies, is intended to counter the seemingly untenable view that every human life, no matter how minimally functional, is of equal absolute worth. The idea is that by blindly valuing the lives of even merely vegetative humans we often do wrong when, for instance, other more highly functioning individuals could be saved by organs or tissues taken from them. From Singer's perspective, what appears to be an admirable moral commitment is in reality an indefensible holdover from pre-scientific religious views. It seems to me, however, that this is not the only way to look at the issue even in the context of modern medical advances. Might we not equally well say, not that the worth of human life varies, but that other things vary? Appreciation varies, for instance. A recent newspaper story presents a case in point.[14] Jeff and Amy Jo Hamon of Blaine, Minnesota, provided eleven years of foster care for an anencephalic girl, Krista Marie, claiming that the experience enriched their lives and that the child showed several kinds of small signs of recognition of their presence in her life. Even if it is true, as Singer says, that no anencephalic child is capable of this (rather than, as Mrs. Hamon saw it, "She may not have had a brain, but she had a soul"), still by Singer's own doctrine of subjective preference, the anencephalic child's life had worth in this family's eyes equal to that of any other child. Appreciation varies. Ask any elderly wife or husband who visits his or her uncomprehending spouse in the nursing home every day. Or ask Katie McCargo who has tended her son every day since he was left in a persistent vegetative state by a 1996 stabbing incident in downtown Boston.[15] Appreciation varies, and capacity to restore function also varies. An ethics student of mine recently shared with the class the story of her younger brother who had suffered from hydrocephalus *in utero* as part of a bad case of fetal alcohol syndrome. Surgery to correct the hydrocephalus caused further problems, and doctors predicted the boy would never walk or talk. Today he does both. In other less fortunate cases, of course, efforts to restore function fail or are beyond the energy and financial resources of family and community to support. But this does not necessarily show that the value of human life varies. Perhaps it shows only that our capacity to foster it in every case is imperfect and varies. Perhaps it also shows that the value of human life is on a higher plane than are the costs and benefits of medical intervention. The fact for example, that you would not trade your eyesight for any amount of money is not falsified by the fact that we would not spend all the resources in the world to cure an individual case of blindness. Vision is precious in a way that transcends cost/benefit analyses, as is human life, and this remains true even though hard circumstances limit our ability to preserve vision, and human life, in every case. In sum, harsh realities can be recognized without abandoning our commitment to the transcendent value of human life.

Singer's second commandment requires that we take responsibility for our decisions and not hide behind what he sees as the specious distinction between acts and omissions. Killing is the same as "letting die," in his view, and we ought not to imagine that in "pulling the plug" on life-support or withholding food or antibiotics we are dong anything different than if we administered a lethal injection. The result of these omissions and acts is the same and so our responsibility is the same. The appeal to "letting nature take its course" is an evasion of responsibility. But is this true? At a minimum it seems we could maintain that killing is the equivalent of letting die *only* in those cases where we could easily save the person's life, other things equal. That is to say, if I can easily save a drowning person without undue risk to my own or another's welfare, and if I neglect to do so, then that does seem to be nearly as bad on my part as killing the person outright. But in the standard kinds of cases of letting die, this not the situation. Other things are not equal, usually, and the decision is an agonizing one of how much of various kinds of costs are to be borne in a doomed effort to forestall the inevitable. Consider the recent case of conjoined twins born in England to a couple from the Maltese island of Gozo.[16] Mary and Jodie were joined in such a way that at most one of them could hope to live beyond a few months. The decision to separate them surgically meant certain and sooner death for Mary (the twin who had an incomplete set of major organs and an incomplete brain), and the decision not to separate them meant certain though later death for both. Removing the allegedly suspect distinction between acts and omissions makes this case all but impossible to discuss, of course. But setting that aside, it is also obvious that there is all the moral difference in the world between Mary's death as a result of no medical intervention, on the one hand, and Mary's death as an undesirable side-effect of medical intervention to save Jodie's life on the other.[17] And it simply is not the case that it makes no moral difference whether we decide against surgical intervention for such a set of conjoined twins or decide in favor of giving them a lethal injection. For the decision against surgical intervention (which was the parents' preference, challenged in the English courts) is precisely an expression of refusal to reject one daughter for the sake of the other, whereas a decision to give them a lethal injection clearly expresses rejection of both. The rejection of *neither* is not equivalent to the rejection of *both*; acts are not *prima facie* equivalent to omissions.

Singer's third new commandment is that we respect a person's desire to live or die. By "respect" he seems to mean "acquiesce in," since his point is that persons (whether human or non-human) have a right to life *and* a right to death, such that their preferences must be granted unless outweighed by other legitimate concerns. Personally, I do not believe there is a right to death corresponding to the right to life, but I do not wish to argue the point here. Rather, I would like to suggest that in the case of a person's desire to die we should show a different kind of respect—not the kind that gives in to the desire, but the kind that listens, appreciates, and takes steps to alleviate the causes of that desire such as pain, loneliness, and fear. As a hospice volunteer for several years in contact with terminally ill patients and their families, I am convinced that the hospice movement is right to hold that the vast majority of patients would not wish to hasten their deaths given adequate pain management, treatment for depression, and simple human companionship. Respect for people's desires regarding death ought always to be subordinated to the fundamental, intrinsic value of human life.

This consideration should also carry weight in another kind of case discussed by Singer, namely, that of women rendered irreversibly comatose by accident or disease who turn out to be pregnant.[18] Such women may or may not have wanted their bodily functions to be continued artificially by life-support technology, but other things equal, the choice seems clear (and many mothers, if not most, would agree) to give the baby a chance at life if possible. Again, the desire to live or die is to be respected, but under the assumption that human life is inherently good. It is only this assumption that gives a proper rationale to the respect enjoined by Singer's third new commandment for the desires of *persons*. For if we can imagine what it is to be a chimpanzee-person, or an extraterrestrial person, this is entirely due to our own inner experience of being human persons, and once again it is the human as such that sheds light on the moral. Of course, for Singer being a person is morally relevant while being human is not, and rights attach only to persons, whether human or non-human. I would say, by contrast, that all humans have a right to life (though not necessarily a right to hastened death) *whether they are persons or not* by Singer's (and Locke's) criteria, or better yet, *because all humans should be considered persons,* humanity being the morally relevant category. It is not that we can scientifically prove they are all persons by measuring brain function, though we can come close enough genetically to proving they are human. But they are *experienced as* being human persons, as the anencephalic girl, Krista Marie, by her foster parents, or the unborn infant by the relatives of its irreversibly comatose mother, or Singer's own mother with Alzheimer's disease by himself.[19]

Singer's fourth new commandment is that we bring children into the world only when they are wanted. Morality is indeed a matter of ideals, not of mere facts about human behavior. Ideally there would be no murders, ideally there would be no war, and Singer along with many others would say, ideally every child would be wanted by its parents or at least by its adoptive parents. Setting aside the permissible remedies in Singer's view, such as abortion and infanticide, let us focus on the notion of a *wanted* child. The idea of "want" is closely related to the idea of "appreciation" used in our discussion of Singer's first new commandment. Many's the child born to parents who did not want it at all at first but grew over time to love and cherish him or her beyond what they could have imagined. No doubt there are also examples of parents whose lives have been made much worse, or at least much harder, due to the decision to keep and raise a severely disabled child. The capacity to appreciate a child, to want it as it is, ranges very widely among humans, all the way from the Hamons who eagerly took in Krista Marie despite being warned that she "had the mentality of a fish," at one end of the spectrum, to those modern marvels at the other end who contemplate parenthood based on a search for the very precisely qualified sperm or egg donor. If we think carefully about the appreciation or "wanted" factor, two points emerge: (1) we ought not to let the value of the life of any fetus, infant, or child be determined by this highly variable and changeable consideration; and (2) we ought to place the actual value of human life as such far beyond any considerations of whether a given life is valued under given circumstances. In sum, the intrinsic value of human life is the reason why wanting children makes sense in the first place, not the other way around. Like your eyesight, though more so, your child is something you would not exchange for any amount of money. This fact, and not "wanting" in the sense of mere subjective preference or desire, is what grounds the wanting and appreciation of children in the proper sense of it. Indeed all children should be wanted, but not in the way Singer recommends.

Getting rid of unwanted embryos is non-problematically permissible for Singer. Because they have no desires and feel no pain, such human non-persons cannot actually be harmed. The argument that they have the potential to be sentient creatures and persons is effective in promoting their protection, according to Singer, only if we assume at the outset, as does the old commandment, "Be fruitful and multiply," that there should always be more humans. But one might easily point out that a former need for increased population is in itself a sign not of the perceived intrinsic value of human life but rather of its instrumentality. That is to say, if Singer means to criticize the traditional sanctity of human life ethic on the grounds of its irrelevance to modern life, he has failed to show that irrelevance. In former times, human lives were used as means to an end, quantity itself increasing the chances of propagating the species and supplying needed labor. Today with the perception of overpopulation human life is cheapened again, in another way, on the pretext of quality of life considerations. But in neither case, so far as these considerations go, has the intrinsic value of human life been addressed or upheld. The advantages or disadvantages of increased population are morally extraneous concerns, in a word, when it comes to the question of what may properly be done to control human population. Clearly not everything we *could* do to reduce the population is something we *should* do. The distinction begins to be properly clarified, it seems to me, by careful respect for the intrinsic value of human life. In a world increasingly home to frozen human embryos whose status nobody quite understands, we would do well to reflect on this difference between *can* and *should*, as regards both increasing and decreasing our numbers.

Singer's fifth new commandment is that we not discriminate on the basis of species. As noted earlier, a large part of his rationale has to do with the analogies he sees between racism and speciesism and between sexism and speciesism. Arguments by analogy have to be closely watched, however, because points of disanalogy are always present and often deliberately obscured. Racism and sexism are often equated, for instance, but they are quite dissimilar upon examination. Skin color in humans is a far more trivial characteristic than sex is, and everybody knows this. For illustration (and another imperfect analogy, to be sure) compare the color of a ball to its shape; you get a far different bounce from a football than you do from a soccer ball, even if they are both green. So if racism and sexism are both wrong, it is for very different reasons. Racism is wrong because it takes a trait which makes no humanly significant difference and acts as though it does.[20] Sexism on the other

hand is wrong because it takes a trait which does make a humanly significant difference (well beyond whether you impregnate or are impreg-
nated) and acts as though it makes more difference than it really does. It
is one thing to invent or conjure up a difference between human beings
(racism) and quite another to exaggerate a real difference (sexism).
When Singer says speciesism is just like racism and sexism, then, what
does he mean? Perhaps the answer would be, a little of both. Like racism, apparently, speciesism according to Singer introduces differences
where they do not exist. Humans are the "third chimpanzee," as he
points out. Like sexism, however, speciesism according to Singer exag-
gerates differences, calling them differences of kind when they are only
differences of degree. Perhaps by thus combining the flaws of racism
and sexism he hopes to illustrate speciesism as doubly wrong-headed.

My suggestion is that we look at all this in a different light. What is
wrong with racism, the manufacture of a significant difference where
none exists, is that it excludes a class of human beings from full membership in the human community. Similarly, what is wrong with sexism,
the illicit exaggeration of an admittedly significant difference, is that it
excludes a class of human beings from full membership in the human
community. Now what is wrong with speciesism? That it excludes a
large and motley class of sentient non-humans from full membership in
the human community? Speciesism cannot really be comparable to racism because it does not consist in the manufacture of a significant difference where none exists. Everybody with any sense knows that there
are huge differences between humans and non-humans in everything
from body hair and bodily adornment to sexual behavior (the ones who
look like us—baboons?—are not the ones whose love lives resemble
ours—parrots, actually).[21] Trick questions about whether you could fall
in love with *Homo habilis* or *Neanderthal man* are beside the point—
who would seriously hold that we cannot know who the dogs are, just
because some of them have been bred to look like rats? The question of
species membership is not obscure, less so perhaps than race or sex in
some cases. But it is morally significant. How significant? Is speciesism,
in other words, more comparable to sexism than to racism, in illicitly
exaggerating a significant difference? The answer again has to be no, I
think, and again the analogy drawn by Singer actually serves to undermine his case. For the differences between men and women are great, as
millennia of comedy and tragedy attest, but we say not so great as to
support the denial of essential humanity to either sex, which would
therefore be wrong. Singer's attempt to displace the arena from humanity (racism and sexism being failures to respect it) to sentience

(speciesism being a failure to respect this) fails entirely because the rationale against discrimination is entirely lacking in the latter case. True,
people of different races and different sexes are all sentient; that is a necessary, though not a sufficient condition of being a member of a human
race or sex. But discrimination against them is wrong, not because they
are sentient, but rather because they are human. Again the human
sheds light on the moral. So we cannot be faulted for discriminating
against members of non-human species on the grounds that in all morally relevant respects they are human, or as good as human, too. They
are not. Speciesism is thus not a moral evil, and not really comparable or
analogous to racism or to sexism at all. True moral evils such as racism
and sexism directly violate human dignity. Speciesism, though mistreatment of non-human animals ought surely to be beneath us, is therefore
not a true moral evil.

The fifth old commandment thus replaced by Singer is one we ought
therefore to reinstate in this or some equivalent form: "Treat all human
life as always more precious than any non-human life." All and only human life has and should have this kind of pride of place in a system of
ethics.

In effect I have been saying that racism and sexism are best seen as vi-
olations of the first old commandment mentioned by Singer, "Treat all
human life as of equal worth." His attempt to cast speciesism as analogous to racism and sexism obscures this fact because he harks back to
the principle of equal consideration of interests, rather than to the first
old commandment's injunction to respect human equality. Thus the
principle of equal consideration of interests, as formulated, understood, and applied by Singer leads to a very different normative picture
of the human world than what has traditionally been endorsed. If we
held to the principle of human equality we would surely not endorse
racism or sexism, but we also would not rest easy about decisions that
sometimes have to be made regarding, for instance, the irreversibly comatose. Singer's ethics, based on the equal consideration of interests,
lets us off the hook in these tough cases, but the old principle of human
equality bids us be mindful that even in a world of modern medical
technology, when the lives at stake are human, we ought to be in awe.
This does not mean that a good person will never pull the plug on
life-support, but it does mean that a good person will never do so without true sadness and regret.

It also means that we ought not to kill one another. Singer had proposed to replace the second old commandment, "Never intentionally
take innocent human life," in the spirit of his principle of equal consid-

eration of interests, for he thought it best to admit that when death is our goal, either acts or omissions may suffice to achieve it, and we bear responsibility for both. In some ways, oddly, this seems to overread human responsibility, just as Jean Paul Sartre does when he says, "I choose being born."[22] Sometimes events and their consequences are largely beyond our control. To withdraw life-support with regret and sadness, or to shoot a dying comrade on the battlefield, is not equivalent to giving a lethal injection to an infant with Down's syndrome or to hitting a terminal cancer patient accidentally with your car while driving drunk. Like the traditional distinction between the wrongness of the act and the culpability of the agent, the distinction between acts and omissions is a natural part of careful, systematic thinking about complicated moral matters. To do away with it, on the grounds that if the upshot is the same there is no difference, is a mistake that will lead to lack of clarity. To do away with the distinction between acts and omissions on the grounds that sometimes it is right to take innocent human life, as Singer does, is a major error that will lead to lack of proper respect for human life and the collapse of morality.

But Singer says the second old commandment "is too absolutist to deal with all the circumstances that can arise."[23] Indeed it is, as every decent moral law ought to be! So is the third old commandment on Singer's list, "Never take your own life, and always try to prevent others taking theirs." Like the first and second old commandments, this one turns out to be flawed under examination by light of the principle of equal consideration of interests. Sometimes people prefer to die, Singer points out, and we should respect that. But it seems to me that even if it is true that we should ultimately respect people's wishes in this regard, which I doubt as noted above, still we should always hang onto the moral awareness that our lives are not just our own, which is the reason behind the traditional injunction against suicide. We are always part of a community of interconnected people, an essential fact of being human, and as John Donne rightly points out, "any man's death diminishes me."[24] Concern for possible scenarios that may give rise to exceptions to the second or third old commandments ought never to displace their essential value to us, namely, that they remind us that in cases of murder and suicide something is always wrong. Singer's replacement commandments, with their neutral-sounding language, appear to remove all vestiges of moral horror, a prospect that should really scare us. Such is the effect, however, of the principle of equal consideration of interests, which flattens out the field of value until everything has merely in-

strumental worth, due to circumstances, as promoting private pleasure
and pain and nothing transcends subjective preference.

Traditionally people have sacrificed themselves, if for no other transcendent value, at least for their children whose historical fragility only
intensified their natural power to focus sorrow, joy, and hope. Though
the usual interpretation of Singer's fourth old commandment has been
something like, "the more babies the better," and though this scarcely
appeals to the twenty-first century, still there is something about the
value placed on progeny that ennobles all our lives. It was fashionable
when I was in college, in the late sixties and early seventies, to say that
nobody should bring children into a world like this, but as time went by,
to their own parents' delight, most of those pessimists more than replaced themselves. Singer himself has children, of course. "Be fruitful
and multiply" tells us, among other things, that children are desirable
because human life is good in itself. Technically, however, the Biblical
injunction (not one of the Ten Commandments, by the way, but part of
the creation story in *Genesis*)[25] was directed at all living creatures. Life
itself is good. But Singer takes "Go forth and multiply" as part of the
sanctity of human life ethic which he opposes.

Traditional Western religion is perhaps more supportive of Singer's
animal liberation movement, and less responsible for the sanctity of human life ethic, than he supposes. In any event, neither the acts/omis-
sions distinction nor the speciesism he opposes are really religious
assumptions at all in the sense of stemming from the so-called Judeo-
Christian tradition. The distinction between acts and omissions is all
over the writings of Plato and Aristotle, pre-Christian philosophers unaffected by Judaism and simply trying to understand human moral life.
Likewise, the human orientation of ethics is unassociated in its origins
with Western religion, being traceable as we have noted to the ancient
Egyptian concept of doing *Maat*, a concept that appears to antedate
even the Egyptian development of theology, let alone our own.[26] The
notion that there is such a thing as right action, that its demands are
binding upon all humans, upon Pharaoh himself and upon the gods,
and that it involves equality of all human beings before the moral law is
very ancient and hardly arbitrary. That a similar but mysteriously more
enlightened concept should hold for all sentient beings as such, as
Singer claims, is wildly preposterous. That it should hold for all "persons" whether human or non-human is perhaps closer to the realm of
possibility—but at a minimum, this is something the human beings will
have to decide.

That any such decision about the ethics of the future is needed now seems highly doubtful, particularly with regard to the complete Copernican revolution in ethics foreseen by Singer. Given the current, pervasive, and all but unnoticed assault on basic human values, I would say the question is not whether we can reform ethics to keep up with the times—will not advertising take care of that?—but rather whether we can persistently value the human because it is human. Many of the pressures on us are against this. To take a seemingly small but telling and perhaps determinative example, an ancient and venerable distinction, one that lies at the foundation of all science and all philosophy, has come close to being erased in our culture. It is the distinction between appearance and reality. Like much of modernity, this distinction and its erasure were prefigured in ancient times and bear revisiting briefly.

At the dawn of Western civilization, in the Greek colonies of Asia Minor, around 600–500 B.C.E., the philosopher/scientists Thales, Anaximander, and Anaximenes, perhaps under the influence of Egypt in her old age, began to speculate about the nature of the cosmos. Things appear very diverse to us, they thought in effect, but perhaps their underlying reality is some unified thing. They and subsequent thinkers proposed cosmic explanations of various kinds, in terms of one or more of the ancient elements—earth, air, fire, water—until argument and counter-argument finally led, in a couple hundred years' time, to the theory of atomism. Ancient atomists held, for a variety of good and imaginative reasons, that all things are made of tiny, invisible, "unsplit- table" particles that move perpetually in empty space. The resemblance between this ancient model and modern scientific materialism is close and not accidental. The ancient atomist, Democritus (c.460–370 B.C.E.), in elaborating the system, was led to declare, "By convention sweet and by convention bitter, by convention hot, by convention cold, by convention color: in reality atoms and void."[27] Notice the subtle passage over time from an attempt to explain the evidence of our senses to the claim that the evidence of our senses is inherently unreal. The reality to be explained becomes mere appearance *explained by* an unperceivable "reality." Thus was born in the West the notoriously powerful reductive analysis: the qualitative world of human sensory experience is *really just* atoms in the void.

Today we have a variety of variations on the theme, "atoms in the void." Photons, quarks, DNA, and so on all play the role of explanatory reality, relegating to mere unreal appearance the myriad qualitative experiences of daily life: light, color, animals, consciousness. What began as an aid to understanding our experience is fast becoming the primary delegitimizer of our experience. What began as the crowning glory of being human, scientific knowledge, has the potential to become a primary usurper of human dignity insofar as it tells us our experience is unreal. How else could Singer and others even consider calling *Homo sapiens* the "third chimpanzee"? But supposedly 98.6% of DNA, as a scientific fact, trumps all personal experience of the vast differences between us and them.

I had said that many forces today influence us against the impulse to value human life because it is human, and many of these pressures come from precisely the most distinctively human activities such as science itself and philosophy. Peter Singer is a philosopher. Time was when to say so would have been *ipso facto* to say that he was a humanist. No more, though as a vestigial reminder, the chair he holds at Princeton is housed in the so-called "Center for Human Values." Singer's brand of analytic philosophy in general, and his preference utilitarianism in particular, seem to regard the human as such as passe, pre-scientific, in Derek Parfit's terms, not even capable yet of real (non-theological) ethics.

Hence Singer's condemnation of human moral intuition which manifests itself via kin preference and the perceived sanctity of human life in such systems of thought as the Western moral tradition. My point, by contrast, is that human moral intuition so far from being inadequate, as Singer claims, is actually absolutely necessary to ethics. Just as human sensory experience of the physical world was indispensable to natural philosophy and physics in ancient Greek times, so even now human moral sensitivity is indispensable to ethics. It is what ethics is *about*. If a system of ethics comes along to discredit it entirely, then so much the worse for that system.

In the first place, human moral sensibility, the capacity for "correct preference," we might say, as distinct form mere subjective preference, is indispensable for recognizing what is right. I do not say it is infallible; that would be another thing. Neither is sense perception infallible, but it is indispensable to physics. The sense of what is right, for instance taking care of your mother in her old age (even if she has Alzheimer's and no longer recognizes you), is so universal that even Peter Singer has it all the while he believes it makes no sense. But it does not have to make sense. It is irreducible in the way that the taste of a pineapple is irreducible. No explanation is needed at all for one who has the experience, as the vast majority do, and no amount of argumentation will convey it to a person who simply does not get it. Or consider the recognition that Mother Teresa was a good person. Any sane human being who knows about her care for the sick and dying in the streets of Calcutta will be moved to condone her acts; that is a matter of moral perception, and without it ethics would be impossible. Singer himself appeals to it in his defense of animal liberation and in his delineation of the obligations of the affluent to the needy. The proposed substitution of mere subjective preference in place of correct moral intuition is inconsistent on his part because of the implicit criterion of correct preference—for the other animals and for the world's poor, which is just his version of the human moral sensibility he claims not to need.

Secondly, being aware of and appreciating one's own humanity is equally indispensable to ethics for it provides the backdrop against which to see the application of moral principles in specific situations. What if I were the one at risk, or whose life and welfare were at stake? This is the foundation of our feeling for one another, and as we noted earlier, ethics would be impossible without it. Even Singer appeals to this when he tugs at our heartstrings for the sake of the higher apes.[28] They're human, he wants us to think. They're not, and we all know it, but insofar as they approach the human we are moved.

The *being* of non-human animals, and perhaps especially of the higher apes, has a kind of intrinsic value, but it must be emphasized that we as humans know and appreciate this fact only insofar as we perceive the intrinsic value of our own human being from the inside. We are not gods or body-hopping extra-terrestrials of some kind that we can perceive this in terms devoid of human content. Nor should we try. Suppose we were to concede to Singer that the source of all moral value is mere subjective preference, and consider the line of argument that would follow. On this assumption, not only non-human but also non-sentient beings could be granted moral value or moral standing. The redwood forests, for instance, or the moon, might be such that to deprive them of existence would be wrong as violating the principle of equal consideration of like interests of all sentient beings, supposing a sufficient number of sentient beings thought so. And perhaps they do in fact think so. It remains true, Singer to the contrary notwithstanding, that in general the value of a being is not strictly reducible to its characteristics, but resides rather as we have seen in its being an object or entity of a given kind. Thus the redwood forests are not replaceable, acceptably to those who love them, by an equivalent oxygen source, say. Nor is the moon replaceable to its admirers by an incandescent light of equal brightness. But the arboreal and lunar realities themselves are required *with* their natural attributes.

Thus we all know that even in a persistent vegetative state a human being is human, hence our tendency to value him or her as such.

Granted that we had far rather have him or her *with* his or her natural attributes, all of them, that we had grown fond of. But identity and humanity are not altogether lost even in those straits. Because we are and
remain human we value them still in their humanity and rightly vener-
ate the physical body we had loved. Even without prior knowledge of
the person, this affection persists and we feel for the unborn infants
of comatose mothers, for the babies with Down's syndrome, for
anencephalic children, the autistic, those in persistent vegetative states,
Alzheimer's patients who have lost their conscious identities, and the
unconscious terminally ill. Let anyone sit quietly for awhile beside even
a heretofore unknown and now unresponsive cancer patient in the
so-called "active dying process," as I have done upon occasion; it is perhaps a criterion of being a normal human being that you can feel in such
circumstances, whether at ease or not, more closely in touch with your
own humanity than at any other time. The deeper meaning of an experience like this seems outside the scope of Singer's ethics. Or rather than
being central, as it should be, it becomes at best peripheral and merely a
matter of taste.

NOTES

1. Singer, *The Expanding Circle: Ethics and Sociobiology* (New York:
Farrar, Straus and Giroux, 1981), p. 71.

2. Singer, *How Are We to Live? Ethics in an Age of Self-Interest* (Amherst,
NY: Prometheus Books, 1995), p. 188.

3. Singer, *Practical Ethics*, Second Edition (Oxford: Oxford University
Press, 1993), p. 94.

4. *Animal Liberation*, New Revised Edition (New York: Avon Books,
1990). All quotes from *Animal Liberation* are from this edition.

5. *Animal Liberation*, p. 3. By any standard, this is an extremely strange
sentence. Both in its original context, and in isolation, it seems to prompt
one to ask whether Singer is saying that "blacks, women, and other groups"
are somehow on a par with non-humans.

6. All quotes are from the 1993 edition.

7. *Practical Ethics*, p. 58.

8. *Ibid.*, p. 19.

9. *Ibid.*, p. 21.

10. *Ibid.*, p. 22 (my emphasis).

11. *Rethinking Life and Death: The Collapse of Our Traditional Ethics*
(New York: St. Martin's Press, 1994). The discussion of the old and new
commandments is to be found on pp. 190–206.

12. *Rethinking Life and Death*, p. 217. See also Peter Singer and Helga Kuhse, *Should the Baby Live? The Problem of Handicapped Infants* (Oxford: Oxford University Press, 1985).

13. See *Rethinking Life and death*, chapter four, "Tony Bland and the Sanctity of Human Life," pp. 57–80. Singer sees the case of Tony Bland, an English teenager who was reduced to a persistent vegetative state in 1989 due to injuries received in a crush of fans at a soccer game, as a test case for the sanctity of human life ethic.

14. Manchester, New Hampshire *Union Leader*, 28 January 1999, p. A8.

15. *The Boston Globe*, 4 December 2000, pp. B1, B4.

16. *The Boston Globe*, various articles in various editions, in particular 7 November 2000, p. A8.

17. For a very clear discussion of this case, including the details of the surgery that was eventually performed, see Benedict Guevin, OSB, "The Conjoined Twins: Direct or Indirect Killing?" forthcoming *Catholic Biomedical Ethics Quarterly*, 2001. The doctors took great care to maintain the bodily integrity of each twin at every stage of the separation, until the last stage when the separation was completed by the clear assignment of her aorta to Jody's body, at which point Mary's death resulted due to her own body's not being able to sustain itself. There is a whole tradition of thought on the general topic of the principle of double-effect, with technical distinctions and terminology that I neither explain nor employ here. The interested reader may wish to look into the matter further under the headings of "natural law ethics" and the "principle of double-effect." Philosophers especially well known for their work in this area are Germain Grisez, John Finnis, and Joseph Boyle, each of whom has published a variety of books and articles, both individually and in collaboration with one another.

18. See *Rethinking Life and Death*, chapter one, "Birth After Death," pp. 9–19.

19. See Michael Specter, "The Dangerous Philosopher," in *The New Yorker*, 6 September 1999, pp. 46–55. Singer is quoted on the topic of the care of his mother: "probably not the best use you could make of my money. That is true. But it does provide employment for a number of people who find something worthwhile in what they're doing. . . . Perhaps it is more difficult than I thought before, because it is different when it's your mother."

20. For a lucid exposure of quasi-scientific foolishness on this topic, see Stephen J. Gould, *The Mismeasure of Man* (New York: Norton, 1981).

21. Many species of parrots mate for life, by and large, with the occasional excursion under pressure. See Thomas Arndt, *Atlas of Conures*, trans. Annemarie Lambrich (Neptune City, NJ: T.F.H. Publications, 1993), pp. 48–49.

22. See Sartre, *Existentialism and Human Emotions*, "Freedom and Responsibility," trans. Hazel E. Barnes (New York: Carol Publishing, 1990), pp. 52–59 (the quote is on p. 58).

23. *Rethinking Life and Death*, p. 192.

24. John Donne, "Meditation 17, *Nunc lento sonitu dicunt, morieris.*"

25. See *Genesis* 1:21–22. "So God created the great sea monsters and every living creature that moves, with which the waters swarm, according to their kinds, and every winged bird according to its kind. And God saw that it was good. And God blessed them, saying, 'Be fruitful and multiply and fill the waters in the seas, and let birds multiply on the earth.' " This passage precedes the creation of human beings. Later, *Genesis* 1:28, God says to the male and female human beings, "Be fruitful and multiply, and fill the earth and subdue it." Singer objects to the idea that human beings are placed in a position of domination (or as Jews and Christians would put it, stewardship) over the other species of living things. Somehow he seems to overlook the fact that God looked at *all* the living creatures and "saw that they were good." See Singer, *Rethinking Life and Death*, pp. 165–169.

26. See Richard A. Gabriel, *Gods of Our Fathers: The Memory of Egypt in Judaism and Christianity* (Westport, CT: Greenwood Press, 2001).

27. See Jonathan Barnes, *Early Greek Philosophy* (Penguin Books: 1987), pp. 252–253. This is comparable to fragment B 125 in the standard Presocratic catalog of Diehls/Kranz.

28. See *Rethinking Life and Death*, pp. 159–163. Singer begins chapter eight with a lengthy "subterfuge," describing the lives of "people confined in a new kind of institution" in the Netherlands. The "people" turn out to be chimpanzees.

Chapter Five

Why Singer's Principle of Equal Consideration Is a Threat to Morality and to Human Values

In one sense it may be true that human beings and the human good are only of peripheral or marginal importance in the grand scheme of things. As we are often reminded, being but one life form residing relatively briefly on a minor planet that orbits a middling star somewhere in a galaxy of stars that is itself but one of thousands of galaxies in the cosmos, we have little claim to centrality or even significance in time and space. Like life itself, though, which defies entropy within a limited sphere, ethics defies human insignificance, and rightly so. The ethical outlook is the view according to which each human being is intrinsically important, no matter how humble, and it is the view according to which the human species as a whole is of transcendent importance no matter how negligible our cosmic impact from the point of view of biology, chemistry, or physics.

THE LIMITS OF OBJECTIVITY AND OF THE UNIVERSAL POINT OF VIEW

Echoing Sidgwick, Singer recommends the "point of view of the universe" as being essentially the moral point of view. This idea is at the heart of his principle of equal consideration of interests, and is to be understood, not as inspiring the conviction that all human beings are equal before the moral law, but rather as placing the interests of all sentient creatures on a par, those of humans included among, but as such no more important than, the rest. As we noted earlier, however, the point of view of the universe is a misleading fiction, because it is only humans (so far as we know—chimps have shown no interest) who could think to adopt it, and because when humans do adopt it they end up denying the very human subjectivity that alone makes adopting the point of view of the universe possible in the first place. You have to have a human mind to do it, in a word, and yet adopting the universal viewpoint is tantamount to denying the importance of having a human mind. This is not a trivial fact, nor the suspect result of logical trickery. The universe really does not care about us, nor about any of the other sentient creatures. The sentient creatures have to look out for themselves, and within that category the human beings have to look out for the human beings. No non-human standpoint, in fact, is one from which human concerns are sympathetically observed. Although the occasional non-human, like the dog Lassie, has saved a human life, and although some of the other higher primates may be fond of us humans despite our intrusive scientific projects, it is distinctively human beings who care about human beings. Just as dogs notice especially other dogs, and cats other cats, so our human sympathy for one another is part of our human nature.

To the extent that adopting the "point of view of the universe" (in Singer's sense of it, consistent with the principle of equal consideration of the like interests of all sentient beings) means subordinating our subjective attachments to our fellow human beings, it is an inhuman point of view. There is no "common good" involved in it, of the kind that can bind human society together at all levels—from the family to the state— because there is no common interest. There is only the sum total of the private interests of individual sentient beings who have nothing in common across the entire range of them beyond the capacity to feel pleasure and pain. But as we have seen above, pleasure and pain have value, not in and of themselves, but only as the pleasure or pain of a specific kind of entity. At a minimum, then, Singer's principle of equal consideration of interests should be restricted to human interests if it is to act as an ethical principle.

Even so the principle fails, however, because the underlying assumption is false; namely, that the more objective our standpoint the more ethical it will be. It is true that being more objective, more detached from our own personal interest, often makes us better appreciate the moral viewpoint. But the opposite also happens. Consider the familiar expression, "a face only a mother could love." By dint of her very proximity and involvement, she perceives a beauty and value that greater objectivity and detachment would only obscure. Or consider a young man in love—"nobody knows what he sees in her." Indeed they do not, because they are too objective. But all of us have to be grateful for people in our lives who have seen good in us that the "impartial observer" would have wholly missed. Granted, sometimes the impartial observer does shed light on the moral aspect of a situation, as when an outsider sees, for instance, that the economic benefits of slavery blind people to its cruelty. But the partial observer also sheds light upon occasion, and so it simply is not true that the more objective we become the more moral we shall be. Perhaps what is morally required is a kind of balance between the partial and the impartial views. But there are problems even with this idea. Parents and teachers, for example, must continually revise the specifics of fair treatment when dealing with two or more very different children, and neither strict equality nor inflexible inequality of treatment will do as a policy over time. Sometimes a little one needs to be indulged, and sometime she or he needs to submit to the group— the impartial, objective standpoint has its uses and abuses, but the partial subjective standpoint does, too. As a teacher or parent, one must have a feeling for both and no absolute commitment to either. It is a gross oversimplification to maintain that the detached, objective, rational mode is moral while the involved, subjective, emotional mode is the opposite. Yet this is essentially what Singer is telling us by founding ethics on the principle of equal consideration of (the like) interests (of all sentient beings).

The essential emptiness of reason considered in itself is at the heart of what should be our dissatisfaction with the purported ideal of objectivity. Without a very rich, if admittedly not crystal clear, concept of *the human* to reason *about*, reason simply goes its merry way, spinning out all manner of claims in the form, "because . . . , therefore . . . ," and nothing intervenes to check the process. This is what we called "calculative reason" in chapter three, and like every kind of reason it needs content to be meaningful. Moral reasoning needs human content to be relevant, and a correct appreciation of the human in order to arrive at moral principles that are binding.

A few examples may make this point clearer. The application of economic concepts is a rational procedure often employed in our day in areas such as medicine and education where it had once been considered inappropriate. Thus the concept of customer satisfaction, so often an implicit part of college admission and retention efforts, is antithetical to the educational enterprise, and threatens to undermine it. For education is not merely a matter of the satisfied consumption of a product—on the contrary, it is a matter, among other things, of growing skeptical of easy satisfaction, of passive consumption, and of popular products. Likewise the concepts of cost/benefit analysis, supply and demand, and marketability, when applied in medicine without regard for human values, yield bizarre results. For instance, when a patient is a so-called "outlier," that is, when his or her condition is unusual and thus outside the mainstream, it is reasonable from an economic point of view not to expend the resources required for accurate diagnosis and treatment. Thus a health maintenance organization medical director some years ago defended the medical neglect of a forty-year-old woman who turned out to have ovarian cancer on the grounds that, "in today's medical care economy we can no longer gear our care to outliers." Leonard Laster, Distinguished University Professor of Medicine and Health Policy, and chancellor emeritus at the University of Massachusetts Medical Center in Worcester, Massachusetts, who recounts this anecdote in a recent editorial,[1] says in reply, "During my medical training, I learned that medicine is all about outliers." At a minimum, medicine is about the individual human patient in all his or her peculiarity, in other words, not about the average customer.

Another example of rational, objective application of economic concepts in medicine is provided by the story of Rachel Sweet, a little girl who needed a lung transplant at six months of age. The journalist commenting on her plight and explaining why her chances of getting a transplant were not good noted that there are fewer organs available for children due to increased use of bicycle helmets, child safety seats, smoke-detectors, and so forth. And he adds, "That depleted organ bank is an unanticipated and underappreciated dark side of the otherwise upbeat trends of declining crime rates and growing acceptance of seat belts."[2] Once we begin speaking of the "dark side" of a "depleted organ bank," can the notions of a "shortage" of human organs and a "demand" for human organs be far behind? But these are human beings, and parts of human beings, that we are talking about. And in fact, a whole market economy of organ transplantation already exists, the idea that one is an organ "donor" giving the "gift of life" being belied by the fact that a human cadaver can be worth as much as $220,000 to for-profit tissue companies, some of whose "products" serve cosmetic rather than life-saving purposes.[3] It is frightening to think where the rational and objective application of economic concepts may take us as new "sources of supply" need to be found to fill "demand."[4]

But equally dangerous are pressures from another direction, namely, the marketability criterion as applied to medical research. It has recently been reported that an international effort is being launched to clone humans in order to "provide children to infertile couples."[5] Either the husband or the wife could be cloned, the embryo being then implanted in the woman's uterus. Dr. Panayiotis Zavos of the Andrology Institute of America and the Kentucky Center for Reproductive Medicine and *In vitro* Fertilization in Lexington, Kentucky, is quoted as saying, "We have a great deal of knowledge. We can grade embryos. We can do genetic screening. We can do quality control." Because the "product" is highly marketable in our society, and the business potentially very profitable, presumably no objective, rational analysis of the economic implications will call a halt to the project, but it hardly follows that the enterprise is morally sound. Assessment of moral value involves more than rationality and objectivity, and more than rationality and objectivity *about* economic concepts. Assessment of moral value also requires subjective engagement with and concern about what is good for human beings. *Should* we focus medical care on the majority or the average? *Should* we have more organs available for transplant, and by what means? *Should* we clone humans, and to what end?

This is not to say that the costs and benefits of medical care should not be considered at all, nor that the plight of those in need of transplants should not concern us, nor that the suffering of childless couples is not real. But in addressing these and similar issues we must put human values first. The marketplace should serve humanity, not the other way around. Yet there is nothing in Singer's ethics, based on the principle of equal consideration of interests, to support this priority. On the contrary, at every turn the ramifications of the principle of equal consideration of interests redound to the benefit of business concerns rather than human concerns. Let us take a look at several of the statements along these lines that Singer has become famous for.

In his *Practical Ethics*, chapter four, "What's Wrong With Killing?" in the section entitled, "The Value of a Person's Life," Singer recalls Locke's definition of a person as a being who is self-conscious and aware of being an individual over time. Then he tells us, in proposing an affirmative answer to the question whether there is special value in the life of a person so defined:

To take the lives of any of these people, without their consent, is to thwart their desires for the future. Killing a snail or a day-old infant does not thwart any desires of this kind, because snails and newborn infants are incapable of having such desires.[6]

Within the context, then, of a discussion about whether killing is wrong, which for Singer involves as we have seen the distinction between persons and non-persons, we see that in effect Singer equates the value of a newborn human infant with the value of a snail. The interests, that is to say, of a newborn human infant are on a par with those of a snail, and not equivalent to those of a self-aware, future-oriented person. Singer is not saying what nobody would believe, namely, that if you told a new mother that her baby had died she would be no more upset than if you told her someone had stepped on a snail. But he is telling us that objectively and rationally, from the point of view of the universe which, do not forget, is the moral point of view for Singer, a human mother's attachment to her newborn baby is subjective and emotional, a matter of her own interests and preferences but not a matter of the actual moral value of her infant.

The question I would like to raise is, would it be a good thing if normal human attachments were to yield to the principle of equal consideration of interests? Would the world be a better place if we believed that the principle of equal consideration of interests sheds more light on moral value and on the moral life than normal human attachments do? That is, should we prefer a world in which moral value is thought to be best perceived from a detached and objective standpoint rather than an attached and subjective one? I think not. The capacity to perceive the human beings who are close to us as endowed with transcendent value and meaning, regardless of their capacities or attributes at the time, is exactly what makes us moral beings in the first place. A human mother (in the biological sense of "human") who saw her infant as worth no more than a snail would be less than human (in the normative sense of "human") and also less than sane.

Singer is also on record as having said,

If a human being is so severely brain-damaged that consciousness is utterly and irrevocably lost, nothing we can do can make a difference to the welfare of that human being. . . . The life of such a being has no more intrinsic worth than that of a cabbage.[7]

This is supposed to be the dispassionate, objective, and therefore morally accurate evaluation in keeping with the principle of equal consideration of interests. The evaluation seems inaccurate to me, though. In a trivial way, the cabbage is worth more than the brain-damaged human being; with a cabbage you can make cole slaw or sauerkraut. But at another, far more important level, the human being is worth more than the cabbage, since the cabbage could not be your father, or mother, or sibling, or child, but the human being could be. To forget this is to make a big mistake. Of course, Singer is interested in the idea that the life of an irreversibly unconscious human being is not perceived as having any value by the unconscious one himself or herself. Therefore, he concludes, it has no more value than the life of any other vegetative thing. This does not follow, however, because the other vegetative things in the world do not bear the kind of relation to the human community that even irreversibly unconscious human beings do. Again, the man in a persistent vegetative state may be your father, the woman in that state may be your mother, such a person may be your child or sibling or lover or friend. To be able to say that their lives have no more value than that of a cabbage, however, may defuse the anguish of deciding what, if anything, to do for them or with them.

Cabbages can be cut up with impunity, and Singer's ethics is designed partly to free us up similarly with regard to certain categories of human beings. The harvesting of organs and tissues for transplant is an enterprise, a for-profit business as we have seen, that suffers somewhat from people's scruples about organ donation and about the removal of life support. The recent scandal at a British hospital in which a pathologist was found to have stripped "every organ of every child who had a post-mortem"[8] shows if nothing else that even when humans are clearly dead and not just irreversibly comatose, their bodies have a kind of value and moral standing among us that means, at a minimum, they must be dealt with respectfully and tactfully. Though we may disagree with the bereaved parents in this situation who insisted on having additional funerals for a child whose organs had been missing, and though we may think parents whose children die will often do right in donating the organs, still we must admit—or risk losing our humanity—that the basic impulse to revere whatever is human is a good, fundamental, and necessary impulse if we are to be moral beings. Without it things human become mere commodities just as things non-human often (though not always) are.

Perhaps Singer would say that ideally the attitude toward a human being who has permanently lost his conscious human capacities ought to be the same as that toward any being that lacks those capacities. As we have already seen, he does locate the value of a being in its attributes and not in the thing itself. Here, in the case of the irreversibly comatose, however, we see the flaw in this implication of the principle of equal consideration of interests. For a being that ought to be capable of consciousness, even if it is not, even perhaps if it never could be (as with anencephalic human infants), is inherently and vastly different from a being like a cabbage from which conscious activity is never to be expected. Let us not lose sight of the very real sadness of that state of affairs in which any human being lacks the capacity for conscious activity, and let us not evade the pain of it by talk of cabbages. The alleged objectivity of the principle of equal consideration of interests, far from putting us in contact with reality, actually removes from consideration much that is important in human reality, and thus in ethics.

Singer has also said, "The fact that an embryo has a certain potential does not mean that we can really harm it, in the sense in which we can harm a being who has wants and desires or can suffer."[9] Setting aside the issues surrounding the concept of potentiality, which are complicated, and which we touched on earlier in our discussion of conception and syngamy, let us note that this statement to the effect that an embryo cannot be harmed is another ramification of the principle of equal consideration of interests. In other words, "harm" is understood wholly within the context of interests, and interests are understood as always involving the present (not just future or past) capacity for pleasure and pain (suffering), for wanting and desiring, and for anticipating the future (depending on the complexity of the sentient being in question). This excludes from the concept of "harm" notions that are ordinarily thought to be closely related, such as those of damage, injury, assault, and violence. But it does seem that one could damage or injure an embryo, and that one could assault it or do it violence. In these senses, one could harm an embryo, even if the embryo has no interests in Singer's sense of the term. Moreover, as medicine advances, it becomes more and more possible to help or aid an embryo, by means of micro-surgery, perhaps. Certainly fetuses are already operated on in the womb, and scientists can make alterations even in one-celled organisms. My point is just that if the concept of helping or aiding an embryo makes sense, then why not the concept of harming an embryo? Granted that Singer wishes explicitly to restrict his claim to the kind of harm that can be done to beings that have present (not just future or past) interests, why the restriction? In this case, again, I think it is because he wants to exclude the *kind* of being from consideration. That is to say, he wants our moral deliberations about it to disregard the fact that an embryo is human.

Moral deliberations ought never to disregard the human, however, because the human good is exactly what moral deliberation is primarily about. Even if Singer were to reply that his system does consider the human good in cases involving human embryos, insofar as it considers the good of the parent organism(s), that is only one side of the situation. And even if we were to concede to Singer that human embryos need not be granted the same consideration as humans who are capable of suffering, it would not follow that their being human is no factor at all. A snail can be injured, a cabbage can be damaged, and a human embryo can be harmed, but unlike the cases of the snail and the cabbage, the harming of a human embryo ought not to be taken so lightly that we claim it cannot occur. Above all, the possibility of such harm ought not to be denied altogether as a way of avoiding our moral responsibility.

Singer is skeptical, of course, about our alleged moral responsibility to embryos, fetuses, and newborn babies. This is in part because, as he says, "I did not come into existence until some time after my birth."[10] In other words, he believes that in the morally significant sense he did not even exist until he had reached the age at which an infant becomes capable of anticipating pleasure and pain. But this presupposes that the *internal* perception of oneself is the criterion of one's existence, which is not a very plausible presupposition. If we really believe that we came into existence some time after we were born, we should check with our mothers, who will assure us (if common sense has not wholly given way to bad philosophy) that we existed and were uniquely ourselves long before we were born. A pregnant mother is aware of the little foreigner within her from very early on, and has a kind of *external* perception of it which, though vague by comparison with what it will normally become, is nevertheless clearly the perception of something human and existing with qualities that can be identified.[11]

Singer's claim that he came into existence some time after his birth and, of course, that this is true for all of us, may be tenable within the context of an ethics based on the principle of equal consideration of interests, but beyond that context it is highly questionable. This is because an ethics based on the principle of equal consideration of interests depends on what may be called a psychological criterion of existence for beings that have moral standing. In the broadest sense of it, this is the criterion of sentience, namely, the ability to feel pleasure and pain. In the narrower sense, it is the Lockean criterion of personhood involving, among other things, what I have called the "internal perception" of oneself as an individual persisting in time. But although the fulfillment of a psychological criterion of existence may be *sufficient* to establish the existence of a morally significant being, it hardly seems to be *necessary* from an ordinary standpoint. Surely an embryo or a human being in a persistent vegetative state may exist even though unaware of that existence.

If Singer had said, "I did not *become aware* of my existence until some time after my birth," that would have been a more accurate statement from an ordinary perspective. The psychological criterion he relies on is certainly a criterion of *knowing* that one exists; it just is not a criterion of *existing*. For the existence of many things is known, not by any being's *internal* perception, but only by some being's (or beings') *external* perception. That is to say, many things are known to exist only from the standpoint of an outside observer. (Of course, many things, too, are known both from the outside and from the inside.) I have suggested above, then, that an embryo's or fetus's existence may be known by external perception to its mother, who counts as an outside observer even though the embryo or fetus resides within her body, because the embryo or fetus is even then a distinct human individual. The fact that it is a distinct *human* individual (who will normally later know itself to be such) is a morally significant fact. And the existence of human individuals, I take it, may be apparent to external perception even when it is not apparent to internal perception—for instance when they are asleep or unconscious, as well as when they have not yet developed consciousness, and when they have irreversibly lost that capacity.

Singer has also written, however, that,

The right to life is not a right of members of the species *Homo sapiens*; it is . . . a right that properly belongs to persons. Not all members of the species *Homo sapiens* are persons, and not all persons are members of the species *Homo sapiens*.[12]

In terms of our discussion above, this means that the right to life (and perhaps other rights) attaches only to those individuals, whether human or non-human, that fulfill the psychological criterion of existence, that is to say, only to those who recognize their own existence over time. The right to life thus provides an instance in which moral standing of a particular type is to be granted to beings in virtue of their having certain attributes and not in virtue of their being beings of a given kind, according to Singer. The idea is that the right to life depends upon its bearer being able to appreciate the right at some level, that is, being sufficiently self-aware and future-oriented to wish to continue living, other things equal. Though there is some sense in this approach, to the extent that systems of morality do generally presuppose conscious participation by those having rights and obligations, it seems to me that the emphasis on the psychological states of those who *have* rights is excessive, and that the psychological states of those who *grant* rights have not received enough attention in Singer's treatment. For Singer's distinction between being human and being a person generates four categories of beings, as we noted earlier: (1) human persons; (2) non-human persons; (3) human non-persons; and (4) non-human non-persons. But it is only human persons, members of the first category, that are capable of making these distinctions and of recognizing rights! This is *not* an insignificant point. The recognition of rights, and the appreciation of the value (even the "sanctity") of human life, can be accomplished only by human beings. From this fact, does it follow that the right to life and the special value of human life should be ascribed only to that relatively small subset of the species *Homo sapiens* whose members are capable of thinking of these things, in other words, who have the relevant psychological attributes? Far from it. Not even Singer thinks that, since he wishes to grant personhood and the right to life to all kinds of non-humans who lack this higher psychological capability. But Singer also wishes to deny personhood and the right to life to those human beings who lack certain psychological capabilities, and this is the focus of my objection.

I think the right to life, and the appreciation of human life that it is based on (given that the recognizers of rights are humans whose inner perception is of human life) are conclusions drawn from a combination of the evidence of external perception and the evidence of internal perception. That is to say, those human beings who are psychologically capable of appreciating the value of human life, and of recognizing rights or judging that rights should be recognized, have a two-fold basis for this appreciation and judgment. In the first place, they perceive inwardly their own lives and the value of life to themselves. This is the evidence of internal perception. In the second place, they know who their fellow human beings are. This is the evidence of external perception, the precision of which varies all the way from the acknowledgement of another human face to the recent scientific finding that any two human beings have 99.9% of their DNA in common. (If we wished to press the kind of quantitative analysis I cast doubt on earlier, we might note that this is fourteen times the degree of DNA affinity between a human being and a chimpanzee.) Thus the appreciation of the value of human life, and the judgment that any being has a right to life, are really based ultimately on human beings' experience of themselves and of each other. The right to life, then, accrues primarily to human beings and to all human beings—not just to those who currently possess the psychological capacity for the internal perception of the value of human life, but to all who are recognizably human by means of external perception as well. The view I here express has two consequences contrary to Singer's view.

First of all, it follows that any extension of the right to life to members of non-human species is done not unequivocally or under obligation, but rather in the basis of analogy and magnanimity. In other words, we see the other animals as like us in a variety of ways, we anthropomorphize them, and we develop sympathy for them as a result. The more like us they are, generally (though we shall note some exceptions below), the more willing we are to share with them something like the regard we have for one another. This may well be a good thing, its increase may be a sign of moral maturity on the part of human beings, and humans in the future may well regard our current treatment of non-human animals as by and large barbaric. It does not follow from this that any non-human animals have a right to life in the same way that humans do; no members of any of their species recognize rights.[13]

Secondly, it follows that the denial of the right to life to any human being, in whatever condition, is unjust. Recall that the impulse behind Singer's denial of the right to life to some humans was a wish to defuse the anguish felt by the parents, relatives, and friends of anencephalic infants, the irreversibly comatose, and those no longer capable of seeing themselves as conscious beings with a future. Though needless anguish is surely not good in itself, it is not good ethical thinking to conclude, because we may sometimes find an action or omission in fact unavoidable that it is therefore right and no cause for concern. Granted, one may feel compelled sometimes to withdraw life support, perhaps even to withhold food and fluids (when death is clearly imminent) or even to terminate a pregnancy (to save the mother's life). Let us not shirk our responsibility for such decisions, nor imagine that we have not contributed to the death of a human being who has the same right to life as any of us. That someone has the right to life, normatively speaking, does not entail that we actually be able to sustain that life, factually speaking. But it does, and ought to, affect the seriousness with which we regard our options and our capabilities in the face of the human right to life.[14]

Finally, Singer is on record has having stated that,

There are other persons on this planet. The evidence for personhood is at present most conclusive for the great apes, but whales, dolphins, elephants, dogs, pigs and other animals may eventually be shown to be aware of their own existence over time and capable of reasoning. Then they too will have to be considered persons.[15]

Together with his statements about human infants and severely brain-damaged human adults this claim yields the conclusion that dogs and pigs (among other animals) may be persons while some human beings are not. This in turn leads to the conclusion that some non-humans have higher moral standing than some humans do. It could be morally worse to kill an adult pig than a human infant, for instance, or to kick a puppy than to kick a severely brain-damaged human being. Granted that we ought not to inflict gratuitous harm on any sentient creature, whether human or non-human, is it really wise, as Singer insists, to leave species membership largely out of consideration when setting moral priorities between individuals and groups of individuals? A recent Associated Press story reports that a group of thirsty monkeys in eastern Kenya stoned a man to death;[16] he was watering his livestock during a drought, and the monkeys managed to kill one of the herdsmen they attacked. Whether the report is true or not, it raises a host of interesting Singerian questions. Could we conclude that the monkeys were persons, capable of murder, or of enforcing justice? Would the cattle count as non-persons, such that the monkeys had a right to the water and the cattle did not? Would the human beings involved have been violating the monkeys' rights? Could the monkeys perhaps have been trying to liberate the cattle from human control, as well as hoping to get more water for themselves? Many more questions could no doubt be raised. From a human moral point of view, however, it seems to me that human concerns necessarily outweigh the concerns of other animals. I do not know whether there in fact are human non-persons, or non-human persons, but if so I think the interests of even the former outweigh those even of the latter.[17] Ethics, again, is a human affair.

In the Caribbean island nation of St. Kitts the vervet population has apparently grown so large that the native human population no longer has any sympathy for the small monkeys who outnumber them.[18] As a result there is a $20-a-head government bounty on the monkeys, and much encouragement of their use in medical experimentation. Animal-rights groups have endorsed a global moratorium on primate research, but the residents of St. Kitts remain unmoved, since they face an "us or them" situation on farms and in the suburbs. From a human point of view, surely human beings have a right to pursue their legitimate interests at the expense of the vervets, even if the monkeys are persons in Singer's sense. And animal liberation activists, especially those outside the situation, ought not to imagine that they hold the moral high ground. Singer's principle of the equal consideration of interests seems to me to be useless in a case like this. The vervet community simply cannot be regarded, from a human moral perspective, as being on a par with the human community, no matter what psychological attributes the vervets have.

Other kinds of situations involving non-human animals may raise other kinds of questions and call for other kinds of answers. ANDi, the genetically modified rhesus monkey of recent fame,[19] and Alba, the genetically altered white rabbit that glows in the dark,[20] represent human uses of animals that may or may not be morally legitimate. But that moral legitimacy or illegitimacy should not be determined by reasoning based on the principle of equal consideration of interests according to which the like interests of non-human and human animals are weighted the same. Our preference for our own kind, that is, for the interests of human beings in pursuing the human good, must be the moral starting point. In Singer's view, though, this bias in favor of the human should be removed by rational, objective analysis of all the relevant interests involved when deciding moral questions. Rationality, in a word, should cure us of it. Let us now attempt to answer his claim in this regard.

WHY EXTREME RATIONALITY MAY MAKE US MORALLY STUPID

How does a person get to the point of making the affirmations we have seen Singer endorse? Briefly, in paraphrase, they are these:

1. A day-old human infant is worth no more than a snail.
2. A severely brain-damaged human being is worth no more than a cabbage.
3. A human embryo cannot be harmed.
4. I came into existence some time after my birth.
5. Only persons have a right to life, not humans as such.
6. Dogs and pigs may be persons, and some human beings are not.

All of these statements sound very odd indeed, and there are others of a similar nature that Singer has made, but for our purposes these six will suffice. How could a philosopher come to make claims that clash so sharply with ordinary common sense?

In the first place, as we have noted above, each of these claims is a rational, logically calculated consequence of application of the principle of equal consideration of interests, as this principle is understood by Singer. The like interests of all sentient beings are to be treated equally (hence the comparison of some human beings to snails or cabbages), and the like interests of sentient beings who have certain specific psychological attributes (who thus count as persons) are always more important morally than the interests of sentient beings who lack those attributes, regardless of species membership. In cases where the claims about snails or cabbages or embryos or non-human persons which follow from the principle of equal consideration of interests seem counter-intuitive, our ordinary moral sensibility must yield to the logic of the principle, in Singer's view. The reason is that the principle is thought to be clearly more reliable than ordinary moral sensibility, such that its logical consequences are more worthy of rational acceptance than are our ordinary views.

Secondly, behind the emphasis on the rationality and objectivity of the principle of equal consideration of interests, there is the desire on Singer's part, as we have noted repeatedly, to defuse the emotional and moral anxiety that accompanies much of our moral decision making. Not only do our emotional attachments produce an unfair bias in favor of those who are near and dear, but our sentimental attachment to the idea of the sanctity of all human life makes it needlessly difficult for us to end the lives of those whose lives no longer have, or perhaps never will have, real value to them. The quality of life ethic advocated by Singer is well served by the detachment he also advocates. Parents may make more rational decisions about when or whether to bring a child into the world, children of aged parents may make more rational decisions about when to end the lives of their parents, and in general, satisfaction of the like interests of persons may be maximized, if we can cease being paralyzed by our very nearly superstitious feelings for members of the species *Homo sapiens.*

Thirdly, there is in Singer's approach perhaps a general distrust of sentiment, particularly of religious sentiment. Like Lucretius (100–55 B.C.E.) in Roman times,[21] and Hobbes (1588–1679) in the 17th century,[22] Singer advocates replacing religious ideas with what he takes to be a clear-headed scientific approach filtered free of the air of transcendence. Rather than replacing religion in the Western tradition with an enlightened humanism, however, as Lucretius and Hobbes had sought to do, Singer wishes to displace humanity from the center of the stage to the periphery. Our high regard for ourselves as "made in the image of God" has been a mistake, he says in effect. To correct this we must relegate the human to one type only of sentient being, and one type only of person. Our special feeling for human beings as such has no place in morality.

To the extent that Singer's ethical theory emphasizes calculative rationality and de-emphasizes emotion, and I think we see exactly this in the six implications of the principle of equal consideration of interests noted above, it is probably not just morally questionable as I have indicated but also psychologically unsound. In any event, the critique of such rationalistic theories currently being launched by researchers in neurology[23] is very interesting and seems to me to ring true.

Ethical theories including Singer's are, at a minimum, guides to moral decision making. According to the neurologist Antonio Damasio there are two main views of how we make decisions, the traditional, "high-reason" view, and his own "somatic marker hypothesis." The high-reason view assumes that,

when we are at our decision-making best, we are the pride and joy of Plato, Descartes and Kant. Formal logic will, by itself, get us to the best available solution for any problem. An important aspect of the rationalist conception is that to obtain the best results, emotions must be kept *out*. Rational processing must be unencumbered by passion. Basically, in the high-reason view, you take the different scenarios apart and . . . you perform a cost-benefit analysis of each of them. Keeping in mind "subjective expected utility," which is the thing you want to maximize, you infer logically what is good and what is bad.[24]

Though not necessarily scrupulously fair to Plato, Descartes, and Kant, so far this sounds in harmony with the calculative rationality of Singer's preference utilitarianism and with his applications of the principle of equal consideration of interests. Damasio continues:

Now let me submit that if this strategy is the *only* one you have available . . . [it] is not going to work. At best, your decision will take an inordinately long time, far more than acceptable if you are going to get anything else done that day. At worst, you may not even end up with a decision at all because you will get lost in the by-ways of calculation. Why? Because it will not be easy to hold in memory the many ledgers of losses and gains that you need to consult for your comparisons.[25]

So Damasio concludes that since we do make decisions fairly quickly upon occasion, and since we could not do so if rational calculation were our sole decision-making method, therefore we must use more than pure calculative reason to decide. In fact, he goes so far as to say, with reference to patients like Phineas Gage and Elliot (a pseudonym) who suffered trauma to the brain:

What the experience with patients such as Elliot suggests is that the cool strategy advocated by Kant, among others, has more to do with the way patients with prefrontal damage go about deciding than with how normals usually operate.[26]

In light of this, and based on his neurological research, Damasio proceeds to propose and explain his "somatic marker hypothesis," according to which normal decision making is aided by learned emotional responses in a process whereby the mind develops in interaction with the world and with the human social environment in a way that leads to healthy functioning and balanced rationality.[27] Without entering into the details of this, which are fascinating, it may perhaps suffice for our purposes to say that current neurological science points to a strong intuitive, emotional, and somatic component of healthy human reasoning. The detached, objective, calculative rational function apparently cannot get its job done without the cooperation of the attached, subjective, intuitive, emotional function. Damasio even suggests that psychopaths and sociopaths are "the very picture of the cool head we are told to keep in order to do the right thing," and that the notorious genocidal episodes of the 20th century are the result of a "sick culture" that visited these pathologies on the general public and could do so again in Western society as currently constituted with its emphasis on calculative reasoning.[28] In addition to the work in neurology by Damasio and others, recent studies of "emotional intelligence" also suggest that human rational understanding of how to navigate in the human and natural worlds is a far richer and more complicated affair than can be captured by the utilitarian model of cost/benefit analyses.[29] Intellect and emotion are not as sharply distinguishable as had been thought.

If there is such a thing as *emotional* intelligence, might there not also be such a thing as *moral* intelligence? And might not an over-emphasis on calculative rationality actually make us morally stupid? The thought, at any rate, that the extremely rational philosopher and the psychopath might both have something unfortunate in common with the pre-frontally brain-damaged should at least give us pause.

Good, intelligent, rational thinking in ethics and moral decision making requires an emotional attachment component. I draw this conclusion not only on the basis of recent work in neurology, which supports it, but also because, as I have argued throughout this book, the fundamental meaning of ethics and morality is to place a special value on the human good just because it is the human good. This in turn means feeling a genuine affection for human beings. Not that we will always be personally fond of all of them, to be sure. But I had said in the conclusion to chapter three that it seems to me that ethics ultimately rests on human friendship. My purpose at that point was to show that from a philosophical perspective we need to be careful to distinguish the various kinds and functions of reason, to insist that ethical theories considered in themselves do not "decide" moral questions, and to admit that reason can legitimately be overruled when it leads us morally astray. It now seems appropriate to add that since healthy rational decision making requires an emotional attachment component it is very important in ethics to ensure that this be the right kind of emotional attachment, namely, an attachment to real human beings. Emotional attachments, in other words, will play a role in our moral decision making whether we like it or not, unless we are to operate at the dysfunctional level of prefrontal brain damage and be unable to make effective decisions. And it makes all the difference in the world whether these are healthy human attachments or mere commitments to principle that disregard their human effects.

This consideration now casts doubt on the highly touted value of impartiality in moral decision making. Maybe kin preference is an indispensable part of our moral development, both subjectively, in that it provides some of the initial emotional sorting functions that enable decision making to come to intermediate and final conclusions, and objectively in that it gives us an enlightened, moral insight into others' kin preferences. Thus, for instance, our special attachment to parents, siblings, and children helps us to decide what to do for them, out of love, and when we see other human beings, even those at quite a distance who are personally unknown to us, we can "feel for" them because we know from the inside how they feel about *their* parents, siblings, and children. It seems more plausible that compassion and kindness grow in this way, than that they result from calculated, rational application of the principle of equal consideration of interests.

Of course, somebody could object that in thus extolling compassion and kindness I have slipped into a "virtue ethics" mode, while Singer is doing something quite different, namely a utilitarian analysis of what our moral priorities ought to be. It is precisely the "moral proximity" of kin preference that clouds our judgment, from his point of view, and leads in the West to the legitimization of "living high and letting die."[30] Singer sets a very high standard of charity toward our fellow human beings in the third world, dedicating 20% of his income to world famine relief, and teaching the basic immorality of indulgence in any kind of luxury or unnecessary consumption while there is any human being in the world who lacks necessities. That this level of generosity can coexist compatibly with the claims Singer has made about the value of the lives of newborn human infants and irreversibly comatose human adults is testimony, however, to the moral emptiness of the principle of equal consideration of interests. Rational application of that principle leads equally in these wildly disparate directions. But my point is that reason must listen, and occasionally yield—from the point of view of any ethical theory—to the promptings of the human heart. A heart in the right place, with an affection and respect for the transcendent value of human life in all its manifestations, though it will not solve all our moral dilemmas (as indeed nothing other than the individual human being on the moral front lines ever will), is a crucial pre-requisite to the moral life. Singer's willingness to do without this bodes ill and threatens our very humanity.

NOTES

1. Leonard Laster, "Why Corporate Medicine Needs Radical Surgery: The Free-Market Approach is Out of Place," *The Boston Globe*, 26 March 2000, p. E2.

2. Larry Tye, "Child's Plight Shows Limits in Organ Donation," *The Boston Globe*, 29 August 2000, pp. B1, B4. See also, Associated Press, Washington D.C., "Change in Transplant Program Cuts Wait for Sickest Patients," *The Boston Globe*, 15 May 2000, p. A12, which includes reference to "a limited supply of donated organs."

3. Associated Press, Santa Ana, California, "Report Says Donated Organs Bring in Big Profits for Companies," *The Boston Globe*, 17 April 2000, p. A7.

4. Singer does address this danger in "Altruism and Commerce: A Defense of Titmuss against Arrow," *Philosophy and Public Affairs* 2, 1973, pp. 312–320. His book, *Marx* (New York: Hill and Wang, 1980) also provides ample evidence that Singer does not endorse the "market society" we have developed in the West, where business values seem to dominate most areas of human life. In my opinion, it is to his credit that he perceives the incompatibility of ethics with business values. The problem is that his ethical theory, considered in itself, provides no means of defending human values against the values of the marketplace. On the contrary, it renders human values more vulnerable to the onslaught.

5. Andrew Stern, Reuters, "Scientists Say Team Will Use Clones to Help the Childless," *The Boston Globe*, 27 January 2001, p. A7. For an excellent discussion of the issues surrounding the idea of babies as products, see Joseph S. Spoerl, "Making Laws on Making Babies: Ethics, Public Policy, and Reproductive Technology," *The American Journal of Jurisprudence*, Vol. 45, 2000, pp. 93–115.

6. Singer, *Practical Ethics*, p. 90.

7. Singer, "The Concept of Moral Standing," in Arthur L. Caplan and Daniel Callahan, eds., *Ethics in Hard Times* (New York and London: Plenum Press, 1981), pp. 31–45. The quotation is from pp. 40–41.

8. Kevin Cullen, "UK Scandal Hurts Organ Donation," *The Boston Globe*, 8 February 2001, pp. A1, A11. Cullen notes, "While some authorities say it is

too early to conclude that the Alder Hey scandal has led many people to re-
fuse to donate their or their children's organs, the anecdotal evidence is
mounting and the government is reacting. . . . Besides compounding the organ transplant shortage [sic], the Alder Hey scandal poses a long-term threat
to research, said Britain's chief medical officer Liam Donaldson."

9. Singer, *Rethinking Life and Death*, p. 97.

10. See Peter Singer and Helga Kuhse, *Should the Baby Live? The Problem
of Handicapped Infants* (Oxford: Oxford University Press), p. 133.

11. It may be more than one "something" in the case of twins or triplets,
or other multiple gestations, but for my purposes the point is the same. We
have here *at least* one human individual, recognizeable if dimly to its parent.
See also our discussion above on the topic of the interval during which
twinning remains a possibility.

12. Singer, *Rethinking Life and Death*, p. 206.

13. No doubt there are non-human animals that may be said to "allow"
others of their species to do certain things, and that may be said to "com-
plain" when they are not allowed to do certain things. But they do not have
the concept of the moral, and they therefore do not recognize rights in the sense
that I intend. Consider a dog who "ought not" to lie on the couch; its understanding is not really that lying on the couch is "wrong," rather being *caught*
on the couch is a mistake. It is quite possible to foresee punishment or reward without having any concept of the moral, and in fact, the moral is first
understood when it is seen to be independent of punishment and reward.

14. For an excellent discussion of this topic, see Roderick M. Chisholm,
"Coming into Being and Passing Away: Can the Metaphysician Help?" chapter six of his *On Metaphysics* (Minneapolis: University of Minnesota Press,
1989), pp. 49–61.

15. Singer, *Rethinking Life and Death*, p. 182.

16. "Monkeys Reportedly Stone Man to Death," Nairobi, Associated
Press, in *The Boston Globe*, 25 February 2000, p. A11.

17. Here my intuitions are at variance with those of Richard J. Arneson,
among others. He writes: "The version of species-partiality needed to solve
the Singer Problem [that no qualities of humans support granting equality to
all humans and granting special moral status only to humans], however,
would have to take the form of a strict obligation to favor one's own species.
What is needed, then, is a morally allowable partiality that takes the form of a
strict requirement: all species members must favor their own species whether
or not they wish to do so. The implausibility of this doctrine becomes evident
if one imagines that it is being applied against humans: the Martian would
prefer to save ten ordinary humans rather than one demented Martian, but
recalling the dictates of 'morality,' he reconsiders, and favors his kind against
his impartial sympathies." See Arneson, "What, If Anything, Renders All Humans Morally Equal?" in Dale Jamieson, ed., *Singer and His Critics* (Oxford:

Blackwell, 1999), pp. 103–128 (quote is from p. 124). The "implausibility of this doctrine" is not at all evident to me.

18. See the story by Mark Fineman of the *The Los Angeles Times*, "Monkey Business Growing on St. Kitts," in *The Boston Globe*, 8 October 2000, p. A14. A vervet is a small monkey.

19. See Richard Saltus, "Monkey is Bioengineered for Study of Human Ills," *The Boston Globe*, 12 January 2001, pp. A1, A25. "ANDi" is a backwards acronym for "inserted DNA"

20. See Gareth Cook, "Cross Hare: Hop and Glow," *The Boston Globe*, 17 September 2000, pp. A1, A36.

21. See Lucretius, *On the Nature of the Universe*, trans. Ronald Latham (New York: Penguin, 1951, etc.), especially Book V, "Cosmology and Sociology."

22. See Thomas Hobbes, *Leviathan* (various editions), especially Part IV, chapter 46, "Of Darkness from Vain Philosophy and Fabulous Traditions."

23. Antonio R. Damasio, *Descartes' Error*. See also, Damasio, *The Feeling of What Happens: Body and Emotion in the Making of Consciousness* (New York: Harcourt Brace and Company, 1999), and Joseph LeDoux, *The Emotional Brain: The Mysterious Underpinnings of Emotional Life* (New York: Simon and Schuster, 1996). In chapter two, "Souls on Ice," p. 25, LeDoux claims that, "minds without emotions are not really minds at all."

24. Damasio, *Descartes' Error*, p. 171. (His emphasis.)

25. *Ibid.*, p. 172.

26. *Ibid.*

27. *Ibid.* pp. 172–201.

28. *Ibid.*, p. 178–179.

29. See Daniel Goleman, *Emotional Intelligence*, (New York: Bantam Books, 1995). Goleman makes use of Damasio's research as reported in *Descartes' Error*.

30. See Singer, "Living High and Letting Die," in *Philosophy and Phenomenological Research*, 1999, vol. 59, pp. 183–187, as well as many other articles and book chapters he has written on this topic.

Chapter Six

On Human Dignity

According to Peter Singer, an ethical Copernican revolution is in the offing, it is inevitable, and the only question is, not whether our traditional ethics will be replaced, but what it will be replaced by. In many ways, however, I think we already live in Singer's world; there is no need to act deliberately to bring it about, it is already here. What we need to do is to counteract the trend before it is too late. On a variety of fronts, moral decisions are being made based on the principle of equal consideration of interests, so that if we look around we can see where this is taking us and why we should not want to go there.

In Wilmington, Delaware, recently a young woman who had pled guilty along with her boyfriend to killing their newborn son in a motel room was released from prison eight months early.[1] Amy Grossberg served twenty-two months in prison, and Brian Peterson, the baby's father, served eighteen months. What this says about our society's estimation of the value of the life of a newborn human infant is something worth pondering. People who murder older human beings do seem to pay a higher price. Perhaps with lighter and lighter penalties for infanticide the practice will become more acceptable, as Singer foresees and advocates, the interests of the parents being more important in his view anyway than the interests of the infant.

In the Netherlands the lower house of the Dutch parliament recently approved a bill legalizing euthanasia, which may make it the first nation to permit doctors to help patients end their lives.[2] Although an earlier Dutch study had found a variety of complications with the physician-assisted suicide process, such as long delays and uneven administration of palliative care (46% changed their minds about suicide, once their pain and nausea were under control), progress in this direction continues, consistent with Singer's recommendations. The right of a person to decide whether to live or to die is a right Singer advocates, as we noted in chapter four. It is not out of place to wonder, however, who really benefits if physician-assisted suicide and euthanasia are readily available. Medical care providers will save money. Families will be spared anguish and expense. Society will be tidier.

In vitro fertilization has been used to allow post-menopausal women to give birth, recently for instance in England where Lynne Bezant's baby was born when she was 56 years old.[3] Though this procedure has many uses, it does seem that the cases of elderly women wishing to become pregnant show how the technology serves and is perhaps driven by a market. Singer's principle of equal consideration of interests paves the way for this sort of thing, namely, by making interests based on subjective preference decisive without regard for questions about whether true human values are supported. What is more important, the desire of a woman past child-bearing age to become pregnant, or the need of a human infant to have a mother young enough to live to see her grandchildren? As a grandmother myself, I do like to think that I have contributed something nobody else could have to my own daughter's experience of motherhood and to my grandchildren. At any rate, this is a value that we probably should not dismiss lightly under pressure from the marketplace.

There are presently estimated to be about 200,000 frozen embryos in the United States, the vast majority of them not "needed" by the "parents" who produced them. This has led to a situation where the embryos are a kind of medical commodity and guidelines governing their use are either unclear or unenforced or both. George Annas, chairman of the law department at the Boston University School of Public Health and a leading medical ethicist, comments, "There are no rules and no one is watching as far as I can tell. So, we're taking a giant step forward, in terms of the technology itself, without having resolved even the most basic issues that it raises."[4] Again, a technology is market driven, and nothing in Singer's ethical theory, based on the principle of equal consideration of interests, provides us with a grasp of the human values involved. Presumably as long as we maximize the satisfaction of preferences for the greatest possible number of sentient beings and persons involved, weighing like interests alike, we cannot go wrong. This amounts to saying that market forces will take care of any problem.[5]

Last year Jack and Linda Nash of Boulder, Colorado, underwent a procedure at the Reproductive Genetics Institute in Chicago to conceive a child whose body would provide a tissue match to help their older child, who suffers from Fanconi's anemia. Without a transplant she was expected to die of leukemia. But the Nash's son was born healthy in Minneapolis, and stem cells from his umbilical cord were immediately used to help his sister develop healthy marrow cells. Arthur Caplan, the well-known University of Pennsylvania ethicist, raises the question, "What about donating a kidney, a piece of lung, or pancreas? How far do you go?"[6] In other words, where do we cross the line between valuing our children for their own sake and creating them primarily as organ and tissue donors for already existing individuals? Even if the particular case of young Adam Nash poses no threat of the disregard of human dignity, given that his parents also want him for his own sake, still the fact that our technological capabilities outpace our capacity to think clearly about the ethical issues they involve is cause for concern. It is especially disturbing to reflect that the ethical issues, whose presence we can all feel even if we cannot articulate them precisely, can be resolved with relative ease by application of the principle of equal consideration of interests. But letting a quasi-quantitative calculus decide seems to threaten our commitment to unquantifiable human values. The intrinsic value of any human infant, the transcendent value of humanity, cannot be reduced to quantitative considerations without terrible loss.

In addition to issues involving medical technology, birth, and death, there are also the perennial scourges of mankind that keep reappearing. Recent studies of the reemergence of slavery around the world and in the United States show that we cannot assume advances in civilization and in technology guarantee similar improvements in human behavior and moral sensibility.[7] Trafficking in women, children, and slave laborers may be the fastest-growing organized criminal activity in the world, there may be upwards of 100,000 slaves in the United States today, and in the Sudan a human slave can be purchased for $35, or slightly less than the cost of a goat. While the topic of slavery is more shocking to us than the topics of physician-assisted suicide, or abortion, or frozen embryos, this is not only because the evil is more apparent or because the subject is less familiar to us. What is shocking about human slavery is that it makes very obvious, in a way that conceiving a child as a tissue match may not quite capture, the sheer horror of treating human beings as commodities. But human beings as commodities, as expendable items whose useful qualities or attributes are the source of their value rather than their simply being human, is the common theme of the situations I have chosen to highlight as being parts of our Singerian world.

One final example may serve to complete the picture. Recently it was reported in *The New York Times Magazine*[8] that business interests are already working on cloning human beings to serve a market that includes gay and lesbian couples as well as infertile heterosexual couples and individuals who prefer not to "take the chance" of ordinary sexual reproduction. This enterprise is supported by large numbers of volunteer surrogate mothers and vast monetary resources, including those of the 25,000-member-strong Raelian cult in Canada, whose founder traces his views on human biological experimentation to an alien abduction experience in which he "learned" that the human race is the experimental creation of extraterrestrial beings, and that cloning is the key to our immortality. The religious angle is perhaps unimportant to our discussion; all it does is serve to explain the motivation of some of the contributors to the wider project of human cloning. What is important to our discussion is the fact that the project of human cloning is so clearly driven by consumer demand. The satisfaction of this demand is yet another and a prime arena for the application of Singer's preference utilitarianism. For the principle of equal consideration of interests will wholeheartedly support human cloning as long as it serves to advance the interests of the majority of those affected. In a world where Singer's preference utilitarianism holds sway there will be no inconvenient obstacles placed in the path of the cloning business, because the principle of equal consideration of interests has no capacity to cope with questions about the intrinsic human value, say, of having one's own unique genetic code, or of not being a carbon copy of somebody else. Will an anencephalic clone in the closet someday be a hedge against depleted organ and tissue banks, shoring up short supplies should the demand arise? Granted that, short of anencephaly, the clones themselves may not be as tractable as their "parents" hope (whose children are?), still our inability to deal with the basic questions raised by the cloning industry, or with the fundamental threat it may pose to our humanity, is not something to be suffered lightly.[9]

In the end perhaps Hilary Putnam has it right when he insists that you cannot do ethics without a "moral image,"[10] without a vision, that is to say, of the world as it would be if things were as they ought to be. Singer's ethical theory lacks exactly that. Although his sense of the obligations of the affluent to the needy, and his compassion for non-human animals, are potentially components of a moral image that would improve our world, they fail in the end because the ethical theory that grounds them as he presents it is so inadequate. As soon as the calculation based on equal consideration of interests is altered, whether by a general change in the majority's subjective preferences, or simply by the numbers of the various parties involved, the obligations and the compassion vanish. The value of the life of a human infant is thus subject to the vagaries of adult preference, as is the compassion we may feel for Singer's (human or non-human) non-persons subject to the vagaries of the interests of (human or non-human) persons, and the obligations we have to our aged parents subject to cost/benefit analyses conducted by the ones who still have "all their marbles"—including competent adult children, health maintenance organizations, perhaps even the state.

Copernicus' model of the solar system may have been a huge improvement over Ptolemy's geocentric model, but Singer's Copernican revolution in ethics, far from being an improvement over the traditional ethics, clearly represents a setback for human values and for our understanding of the human good. To the extent that his preference utilitarianism has already caught on (and it does seem to be exquisitely well-adapted to capitalism and to the values of the marketplace), we can already see where it leads, and we can already see the need to reconsider and to reassert our humanity. Human dignity is not like the earth, which can be displaced by a heliocentric model of the solar system without losing its identity as a habitable planet. Human dignity depends for its preservation on the uniquely human view, which we relinquish at our peril, and which we have an obligation in justice to bequeath intact to future generations.

NOTES

1. Associated Press, "Woman Who Killed Baby Wins Release," *The Boston Globe*, 10 May 2000, p. A16.

2. Anthony Deutsch, Associated Press, "Netherlands Parliament Advances Doctor-Assisted Suicide," *The Boston Globe*, 29 November 2000, p. A17.

3. Kevin Cullen, "Test-tube Pregnancy at 56 Rekindles Debate in Britain," *The Boston Globe*, 23 January 2001, p. A9.

4. Adam Pertman, "The Future On Ice: Unwanted Human Embryos Provide the Raw Material for a Troubling New Form of Adoption," *The Boston Globe*, 8 August 2000, pp. E1, E4.

5. It is not enough for the author of an ethical theory to be opposed to market forces (as Singer says he is). Rather the ethical theory itself must be constructed in such a way as to provide a defense of human values against business values, something that in my opinion Singer's ethical theory does not do.

6. See Andrew Stern, Reuters, "Ethics of Cell Transfer Debated," *The Boston Globe*, 4 October 2000, p. A3. See also, Associated Press, Minneapolis, "In Medical First, Embryo Created for Sibling Transplant," *Manchester New Hampshire Union Leader*, p. D10, and George Annas, "Conceiving One Child to Save Another," *The Boston Globe*, 15 October 2000, pp. C1–2.

7. See Emma Dorothy Rheinhardt and Charles Jacobs, "A Secret Slave Trade Survives in U.S.," *The Boston Globe*, 27 November 2000; William Raspberry, "Heroism, Slavery, and Gum Arabic," *The Boston Globe*, 4 October 2000, p. A21; and Axel Bugge, Reuters, "Crime Gangs Revive Slave Trade, UN Says," *The Boston Globe*, 29 November 2000, p. A15.

8. Margaret Talbot, "Lab of the Human Clones: A Desire to Duplicate," *The New York Times Magazine*, 4 February 2001, pp. 40–45, 67–8.

9. One of the basic questions raised by the prospect of cloning human beings is what to do about the (perhaps majority of) resulting individuals that have gross abnormalities. See Michael C. Brannigan, ed., *Ethical Issues in Human Cloning* (New York: Seven Bridges Press, 2001), which includes articles by George J. Annas, Richard Dawkins, Stephen Jay Gould, Gregory E. Pence, and others.

10. Putnam, *The Many Faces of Realism: The Paul Carus Lectures* (LaSalle, Illinois: Open Court, 1987). See especially Lecture III, "Equality and Our Moral Image of the World," pp. 41–62. Putnam holds that we need a philosophical anthropology, an image of human nature, in order to fend off the situation depicted in Aldous Huxley's *Brave New World*.

Select Bibliography

Aristotle. *The Ethics of Aristotle: The Nicomachean Ethics.* Trans. J.A.K. Thomson, rev. Hugh Tredennick, intro., Jonathan Barnes. London: Penguin, 1976.

Arras, John D. and Bonnie Steinbeck, eds. *Ethical Issues in Modern Medicine,* fifth edition. Mountainview, CA: Mayfield Publishing Company, 1999.

Bentham, Jeremy. *Introduction to the Principles of Morals and Legislation.* New York: Hafner, 1948.

Brannigan, Michael C., ed. *Ethical Issues in Human Cloning.* New York: Seven Bridges Press, 2001.

Brentano, Franz. *The Origin of Our Knowledge of Right and Wrong.* Trans. Chisholm and Schneewind. London: Routledge and Kegan Paul, 1969.

———. *Psychology From an Empirical Standpoint.* Trans. Rancurello, Terrell and MacAllister. New York: Humanities Press, 1973.

———. *The Foundation and Construction of Ethics.* Trans. and ed., Elizabeth Schneewind. New York: Humanities Press, 1973.

Caplan, Arthur L., and Daniel Callahan, eds. *Ethics in Hard Times.* New York and London: Plenum Press, 1981.

Caputo, John D. *Against Ethics.* Bloomington and Indianapolis: Indiana University Press, 1993.

Cavalieri, Paola, and Peter Singer, eds. *The Great Ape Project: Equality Beyond Humanity.* New York: St. Martin's Griffin, 1993.

Chisholm, Roderick M. *Brentano on Intrinsic Value.* Cambridge: Cambridge University Press, 1986.

———. *On Metaphysics.* Minneapolis: University of Minnesota Press, 1989.

Damasio, Antonio R. *Descartes' Error: Emotion, Reason, and the Human Brain.* New York: Avon Books, 1994.

———. *The Feeling of What Happens: Body and Emotion in the Making of Consciousness.* New York: Harcourt Brace and Company, 1999.

Darwin, Charles. *The Descent of Man.* Intro. H. James Birx. New York: Prometheus Books, 1998.

Diamond, Jared. *The Rise and Fall of the Third Chimpanzee.* New York: HarperCollins, 1991.

Dombrowski, Daniel A. *Babies and Beasts: The Argument from Marginal Cases.* Urbana and Chicago: University of Illinois Press, 1997.

Fehige, Christoph, and Ulla Wessels. *Preferences.* Berlin and New York: Walter de Gruyter, 1998.

Frey, R.G. *Rights, Killing and Suffering.* Oxford: Blackwell, 1983.

Gabriel, Richard A. *Gods of Our Fathers: The Memory of Egypt in Judaism and Christianity.* Westport, CT: Greenwood Press, 2001.

Goleman, Daniel. *Emotional Intelligence.* New York: Bantam Books, 1995.

Gould, Stephen Jay. *The Mismeasure of Man.* New York: Norton, 1981.

———. *Full House: The Spread of Excellence from Plato to Darwin.* New York: Harmony Books, 1996.

Hare, R.M. *Freedom and Reason.* London: Oxford University Press, 1963.

———. *Moral Thinking: Its Levels, Method, and Point.* Oxford: Clarendon Press, 1981.

———. *Objective Prescriptions and Other Essays.* Oxford: Clarendon Press, 1999.

Hobbes, Thomas. *Leviathan.* Parts I and II. Indianapolis: Bobbs-Merrill, 1958.

Hume, David. *A Treatise of Human Nature.* Analytical Index by L.A. Selby-Bigge. Second Edition, revised and with notes by P.H. Nidditch. Oxford: Oxford University Press, 1978.

Jamieson, Dale, ed. *Singer and His Critics.* Oxford: Blackwell, 1999.

Kant, Immanuel. *Foundations of the Metaphysics of Morals.* Trans. Lewis White Beck. Indianapolis: Bobbs-Merrill, 1959.

———. *Critique of Practical Reason, and Other Writings in Moral Philosophy.* Trans., ed., and intro., Lewis White Beck. New York: Garland, 1976.

Leahy, Michael P.T. *Against Liberation: Putting Animals in Perspective.* New York: Routledge, 1991.

LeDoux, Joseph. *The Emotional Brain: The Mysterious Underpinnings of Emotional Life.* New York: Simon and Schuster, 1996.

Lucretius. *On the Nature of the Universe.* Trans., Ronald Latham. New York: Penguin, 1951.

MacIntyre, Alasdair C. *Dependent Rational Animals: Why Human Beings Need the Virtues.* Chicago: Open Court, 1999.

Magel, Charles. *Keyguide to Information Sources in Animal Rights.* London: Mansell, 1989.

Mill, John Stuart. *Utilitarianism.* Ed. and intro., George Sherr. Indianapolis: Hackett, 1979.

Mirandola, Pico della. *On the Dignity of Man, On Being and the One, Heptaplus.* Trans. Walles, Miller, and Carmichael. Indianapolis: Bobbs-Merrill, 1965.

Moreland, J.P., and Scott B. Race. *On the Nature and Ethical Treatment of Human Persons.* Downer's Grove, IL: Intravarsity Press, 2000.

Nagel, Thomas. *The View From Nowhere.* Oxford: Oxford University Press, 1986.

Noddings, Nel. *Caring: A Feminine Approach to Ethics and Moral Education.* Berkeley and Los Angeles: University of California Press, 1984.

Parfit, Derek. *Reasons and Persons.* Oxford: Clarendon Press, 1984.

Putnam, Hilary. *The Many Faces of Realism: The Paul Carus Lectures.* Lasalle, IL: Open Court, 1987.

Searle, John R. *Mind, Language, and Society.* New York: Basic Books, 1998.

Sidgwick, Henry. *The Methods of Ethics.* Seventh Edition. London: Macmillan, 1907.

Singer, Peter. *Marx.* New York: Hill and Wang, 1980.

———. *The Expanding Circle: Ethics and Sociobiology.* New York: Farrar, Straus and Giroux, 1981.

——— and Helga Kuhse. *Should the Baby Live? The Problem of Handicapped Infants.* Oxford: Oxford University Press, 1985.

———. *Animal Liberation.* New Revised Edition. New York: Avon Books, 1990.

———. *Practical Ethics.* Second Edition. Cambridge: Cambridge University Press, 1993.

———. *Rethinking Life and Death: The Collapse of Our Traditional Ethics.* New York: St. Martin's Press, 1994.

———. *How Are We to Live? Ethics in an Age of Self-Interest.* Amherst, NY: Prometheus Books, 1995.

———. *Ethics Into Action: Henry Spira and the Animal Rights Movement.* Lanham, MD: Roman and Littlefield, 1998.

Spencer, Herbert. *The Principles of Ethics.* Vols. I and II. Indianapolis: Liberty Classics, 1978.

Taylor, Angus. *Magpies, Monkeys and Morals: What Philosophers Say About Animal Liberation.* Peterborough, Ontario: Broadview Press, 1999.

van Ingen, John. *Why Be Moral?* New York: Peter Lang, 1994.

Wells, H.G. *The Island of Dr. Moreau,* in *H.G. Wells: Three Novels.* London: Heinemann, 1963.

Westermarck, Edward. *The Origin and Development of the Moral Ideas.* London: Macmillan, 1908.

Wilson, Edward O. *Sociobiology: The New Synthesis.* Cambridge, MA: Belknap Press of Harvard University Press, 1975.

————. *On Human Nature.* Cambridge, MA: Harvard University Press, 1978.

Index

About the Author

SUSAN LUFKIN KRANTZ is Professor of Philosophy at St. Anselm College, Manchester, NH. She has translated and edited the English edition of Brentano's lectures on natural theology entitled *On the Existence of God* (1987).